Simple Skin Surgery

SUSAN BURGE
DM, FRCP
Consultant Dermatologist
Stoke Mandeville Hospital NHS Trust
Aylesbury, Bucks

D0552412

GRAHAM COLVER
DM, FRCP
Consultant Dermatologist
Royal Hospital
Chesterfield, Derbyshire

RUTH LESTER
MB, ChB, FRCS
Consultant Plastic Surgeon
Sandwell General Hospital
Sandwell Healthcare NHS Trust
West Midlands

SECOND EDITION

WILEY

Published by John Wiley & Sons, Hoboken, NJ

For general information on our other products and services, please contact our Customer Care Department within the United States at 800-762-2974, outside the United States at 317-572-3993 or fax 317-572-4002.

For more information about Wiley products, visit our website at www.wiley.com.

ISBN 0-86542-690-2

Library of Congress
Cataloging-in-Publication Data

Burge, S.M. (Susan M.)
    Simple skin surgery/
    Susan Burge, Ruth Lester. — 2nd ed.
        p.   cm.
    Includes bibliographical references
    and index.
    ISBN 978-0-86542-690-2
    1. Skin — Surgery.
    I. Lester, Ruth. II. Title.
    [DNLM: 1 Skin — surgery — handbooks.
    WR 39 B954s 1996]
    RD520. B865   1996
    617.4'77059 — dc20
    DNLM/DLC
    for Library of Congress   95-50692
                                       CIP

Contents

Preface

The second edition of this book is still a very practical guide to the simple surgical techniques which may be used to treat skin lesions. Now most GPs have access to excellent facilities for surgery, more and more minor surgery is being carried out in primary care. The book is written for the GP or hospital trainee embarking on skin surgery.

We have expanded some sections but simplified others. The addition of colour illustrations will help clinicians to differentiate benign and malignant skin tumours. Techniques such as punch biopsy, excision, curettage, cautery, diathermy and cryosurgery are described and clearly illustrated. We have included a new chapter in which we discuss the special techniques used for managing problems such as ingrowing toenails, acne cysts and chondrodermatitis nodularis chronica helicis. We also discuss wound problems, how they can be avoided and how to treat them if they arise. Although this is still primarily a surgical book, we have included a short section on the topical treatments used for some skin lesions.

Introduction

Who should be doing simple skin surgery?

Every patient has the right to expect an appropriate level of competence from the doctor who operates on him. Although every doctor has a surgical qualification, e.g. bachelor of surgery, clearly this does not give the doctor the right to perform any operation of his choice.

Generally, in a hospital setting, simple skin surgery will be performed in accident and emergency departments, dermatology outpatient clinics or in the day theatres. There will be supervision and training to the point where the practitioner becomes confident and competent to operate alone. The Royal Colleges are working on logbook systems to keep track of an individual's progress with reference to the number and type of operations performed and the level of supervision.

In general practice the situation is somewhat different. Here some doctors have considerable surgical experience while others have only surgical housejobs behind them. Various regulations and recommendations apply to general practitioners (GPs) who have the interest and skills to perform surgery. To claim a fee the GP must be included in the Family Health Service Authority's (FHSA) minor surgery list. The fee is paid for sessions provided for his own patients or for those of his partners. The following procedures, which attract a fee, relate to the skin: incision of abscesses and cysts; excision of cysts, lipomas and dermal lesions, e.g. melanocytic naevi and dermatofibromas; curettage of viral and seborrhoeic warts; cryosurgery of warts and molluscum contagiosum. Doctors who want to do minor surgery must apply to the FHSA and fulfil the qualifying criteria.

Guidelines from the General Medical Services Committee on training for and practice of minor surgery

The General Medical Services Committee (GMSC) together with: the Royal College of General Practitioners; the Royal

College of Surgeons of England; the Royal College of Surgeons of Edinburgh; the British Society for Dermatological Surgery and the Joint Committee on Postgraduate Training for General Practice have made joint recommendations concerning minor surgery in general practice. They are drawn up to ensure an appropriate standard of care. They point out that before 1990 about 25% of GPs carried out minor surgical procedures but now nearly 75% of GPs are on minor surgery lists.

A summary of these guidelines follows.

Workshops

Many practitioners will wish to undertake training either because they have not previously performed this work or to familiarize themselves with new ideas and techniques. Doctors on the vocational training scheme should be able to attend courses in their area which are approved for a Postgraduate Education Allowance (PGEA). Practical techniques should be demonstrated and taught by experienced doctors who are currently using them.

Initial clinical training

All doctors should have gained supervised clinical experience either in primary or secondary care. Doctors should attend a minimum of three practical sessions with accredited teachers and should obtain a statement of satisfactory performance after each.

Extended supervised experience

Extended attachments to work in specialized departments or with experienced colleagues should be encouraged and recognition of this experience considered for a PGEA.

Content of workshops

These should consist of the equivalent of two full days and contain a practical component which utilizes simulated tissue. The course should cover premises and equipment, rules and regulations and medico-legal aspects. The anatomy of the skin and the pathology and diagnosis of skin lesions must be discussed. Practical techniques must be covered in detail including the choice of instruments and the principles of suturing, local anaesthesia, infection control and resuscitation.

The role of audit should be covered with reference to clinical records, patient satisfaction and diagnostic accuracy.

Guidelines for surgical management of common skin conditions in general practice

These guidelines were drawn up in December 1994 by the British Society for Dermatological Surgery (affiliated to the British Association of Dermatologists) with the Royal College of General Practitioners.

Surgical treatment should not be attempted without a clinical diagnosis. If the diagnosis is not known it is impossible to know whether surgery is appropriate or necessary.

If surgery is for cosmetic reasons the optimal cosmetic result must be achieved. Unsightly scars are a common cause for complaint and expectations are higher when the treatment is cosmetic. Confident diagnosis and reassurance are often the treatment of choice.

Diagnostic procedures
1 Biopsy of rashes or tumours prior to referral to a dermatologist is not necessary.
2 Biopsy of a rash is often unhelpful unless:
   (a) there is a good differential diagnosis;
   (b) the correct biopsy site has been selected;
   (c) the result can be discussed with a pathologist.

Appropriate surgical procedures
1 Shave excision for lightly pigmented moles.
2 Snip/cautery for skin tags.
3 Curettage for seborrhoeic and filiform warts.
4 Cryosurgery for warts, keratoses, molluscum contagiosum.
5 Excision of cysts, lipomas and dermatofibromas.
6 Lateral chemical matricectomy for ingrown toenails.

3

Viral warts—points to remember
1 80 per cent respond to paints within 100 days.
2 Plane warts on the face are best left untreated.
3 Unresponsive warts may be treated with cryosurgery.
4 Cryosurgery is painful and badly tolerated in children.
5 Mosaic plantar warts rarely respond to cryosurgery.
6 Curettage may result in scarring.

Caution
Elliptical excision of benign moles often leaves noticeable scarring especially on the upper trunk, shoulders and the tops of the arms. Beware of surgery in these keloid-prone sites. Consider carefully whether a benign mole needs to be excised.

Elliptical excision of seborrhoeic warts is inappropriate; curettage and cautery are the treatment of choice. Submit all specimens for histology.

• Avoid using braided silk sutures which leave stitch marks unless removed early.
• Avoid using alcohol-based antiseptic solutions with diathermy or cautery, as they are a fire hazard.
• Avoid treating skin malignancies unless experienced in the field. They require adequate lateral and deep margins of excision.
• Avoid the incisional biopsy of moles. Refer patients with suspicious moles. These lesions should always be excised with a defined margin along the correct anatomical axis.

Simple treatments for skin tumours
Patients with benign skin lesions demand treatment primarily because they do not like the appearance of their skin. If the doctor plans to remove a benign lesion, he must ensure that the final result does not look worse than the original lesion and that the possible outcome of treatment should be discussed with the patient. However, if the lesion is malignant, the aim of the treatment must be complete destruction or removal of the tumour. Malignancies in difficult areas (see Chapter 5), e.g. the

alar bases or the inner canthi, need to be adequately excised and therefore should be referred directly for reconstructive surgery. Tumours close to the eyelids or on the vermilion border of the lip should only be treated by a surgeon familiar with the specialized surgical techniques needed in these areas.

There are many methods of treating skin tumours and each technique has its own advantages and disadvantages. The method chosen depends not only on clinical parameters, but also on patient preference, the skills of the doctor, and the availability of equipment. It may be helpful to plan the treatment of difficult cases in a 'combined clinic' which is run by a multi-disciplinary team (dermatologists, plastic surgeons and radiotherapists). Most of the techniques listed in Table 1.1 below are described in more detail in subsequent chapters.

Safe practice and sterility

Principles
The advent of HIV infection has made people look carefully at their clinical practice. The principles are no different from those that have always governed good clinical practice. It is natural to be especially vigilant if a patient is known to be HIV or HBsAg positive but in reality the surgeon should always take the same precautions.

Wound infection is mainly associated with dead tissue, haematomas and foreign bodies, but the skin has a good blood supply and the risk of infection is low (see Chapter 9). The skin should be handled gently and as little as possible. Wounds should never be closed under tension. Cautery or diathermy must be kept to a minimum. Dead spaces should be closed with subcutaneous sutures using as little suture material as possible.

Preoperative assessment
Information should be sought about diabetes, bleeding tendencies, pacemakers, pregnancy, hepatitis or HIV, etc.

Table 1.1 Treatments for skin tumours.

Condition	Treatment
Benign	
Seborrhoeic wart (seborrhoeic keratosis)	Shave, curette, cryosurgery
Viral wart	Cryosurgery, curette, diathermy
Cellular (intradermal) naevus	Shave, excise
Pyogenic granuloma	Excise, curette and cautery or diathermy
Spider angioma	Diathermy, electrolysis
Epidermal and pilar cysts	Excise
Chondrodermatitis nodularis chronica helicis	Excise, intralesional steroid after biopsy
Dermatofibroma	Excise
Kerato-acanthoma	Excise, biopsy and curette, radiotherapy
Premalignant	
Solar keratosis	Cryosurgery, excise, curette
Bowen's disease	Biopsy and cryosurgery, excise, curette and cautery
Malignant	
Basal cell carcinoma	
nodular	Excise, radiotherapy
superficial	Excise, cryosurgery, curette, radiotherapy,
morphoeic	Excise, radiotherapy
Squamous cell carcinoma	Excise, radiotherapy
Malignant melanoma	Excise

Counselling
The patient should know the type of procedure to be performed and alternative treatments and that it will be done in a operating theatre under local anaesthetic. Any likely complications should be discussed.

Consent
This follows naturally after counselling.

Facilities
A dedicated treatment area is essential. Flaps and grafts should be performed in a standard area for day-case surgery. Minor

procedures are safely performed in outpatient or GP surgery accommodation. There should always be space to move and good lighting.

Skin preparation

1 Visible dirt should be washed off with a detergent. The skin should be cleaned with a quick-acting antiseptic, e.g. chlorhexidine solution. It is not essential to clean the skin with antiseptics before cryosurgery, as the intense cold kills any microflora.

2 After washing the skin, the lesions should be surrounded with sterile drapes. A window can be cut in the centre of a sterile disposable paper towel and this simply placed over the area to be treated.

3 Do not shave hair-bearing skin unless absolutely essential, as this increases the infection rate by increasing the number of organisms on the skin surface. Cleaning with detergents and clipping the hair back should usually suffice.

Preparation of the surgeon

1 'Scrubbing up' is not essential or even desirable. A 5 min scrub merely contaminates the skin with bacteria released from the hair follicles. Visible dirt or blood should be removed, the finger nails cleaned and two simple washes in running water, using 4% chlorhexidine detergent solution (Hibiscrub) or 10% povidone-iodine surgical scrub (Betadine), are adequate. In this way transient flora are removed and residues of the antiseptic continue to act against resident bacteria.

2 Gloves protect the patient and surgeon and should be worn for all procedures. Double gloving provides significant protection from needlestick injuries. Masks are of unproven value but a splash mask may keep tiny droplets of blood out of the surgeon's eyes. Gowns help to protect the surgeon's clothes but plastic aprons are equally as good.

Equipment

See Table 1.2, page 8.

Table 1.2 Essential and optional equipment.

Essential	Optional
THE ROOM (see Fig. 3.1a)	
An examination couch with adjustable backrest	Theatre table
A stool for the surgeon	
Good lighting: anglepoise lights	Overhead theatre lights
EQUIPMENT—PREOPERATIVE PREPARATION	
Autoclave for steam sterilization or electric oven for dry heat sterilization	
Skin preparation:	
chlorhexidine solution	
chlorhexidine detergent (Hibiscrub)	
surgical gloves	
Sterile paper towels:	Re-usable drapes
a window can be cut in the centre and the towel placed over the lesion	
Skin markers:	Sterile pen and Indian ink
gentian violet and pointed orange stick	
skin marker pen	
indelible felt-tip pen	
ANAESTHETIC (see Fig. 3.1b)	
Disposable syringes 2 ml, 5 ml	Dental syringe and fine needles
fine needles	Dental syringe vials
Lignocaine:	
1% and 2% plain and with adrenaline 1 : 100 000 or 1 : 200 000	
INSTRUMENTS (see Fig. 2.1b)	
Scalpel blades:	
No. 15 for excision	
No. 22 for shave biopsy	
scalpel handle	
Forceps:	
fine-toothed (e.g. Adson–Brown)	
non-toothed	

Continued

Table 1.2 *Continued*

Essential	Optional

Skin hook:
can easily be constructed by
   pushing a sterile needle onto a
   sterile moistened cotton wool bud
   on an orange stick. Bend the needle
   into a curve.	

Scissors:
curved pointed iris scissors
blunt straight scissors
Needle holders
Small artery clamps
Various sizes of absorbable and
   non-absorbable sutures attached
   to needles (see Chapter 5)
	Skin punch for biopsies,
	   3 mm and 4 mm
	Sharp ring curettes in
	   various sizes

HAEMOSTASIS
Gauze swabs
30–50% aluminium chloride
   in alcohol or Monsel's solution
   (67.5% basic ferric sulphate)
	Hyfrecator
	Electrocautery
	Diathermy
	Bipolar electrocoagulation
	Cryosurgery gun
	Supply of liquid nitrogen
	Silver nitrate sticks

DRESSINGS
Steri-strips
Compound Benzoin tincture BP
   (Friar's balsam) for sticking
   plaster to skin
Elastoplast
Micropore
Gauze
Jelonet
	OpSite

HISTOPATHOLOGY
Specimen pots
 	
Fixative:
   10% buffered formalin
	EM fixative 4%
	   glutaraldehyde
	Fixative or liquid nitrogen
	   to store specimens for
	   immunohistology

Care of instruments

Dried pus or blood on an instrument may contain potentially dangerous organisms, so instruments should always be washed before sterilizing either in an autoclave or in an electric oven. Water boiling at atmospheric pressure will not sterilize because a temperature above 100°C is required to ensure destruction of bacterial spores by moist heat. Instruments should not be left lying in a 'sterilizing solution' which may be contaminated, but should be kept in sterile packs.

Common Skin Tumours

A differential diagnosis of all skin tumours is beyond the scope of this book, but we include a summary of the features of tumours which we envisage being treated by simple surgical procedures.

Acquired melanocytic naevi

Pigmented lesions

These are frequently a cause of anxiety. Benign lesions are usually uniformly pigmented, with a smooth outline and symmetrical contour. Irregularity in pigmentation, margin or thickness suggests malignancy (Fig. 2.1 and Table 2.1). The depth of colour is not an important distinguishing feature.

The features of acquired melanocytic naevi (Plate 2.1) change with age. Children and young adults may have many flat brown 'junctional' naevi in which the naevus cells are distributed along the junction of the epidermis and dermis. As the naevi 'mature', the naevus cells descend into the dermis and the lesion becomes

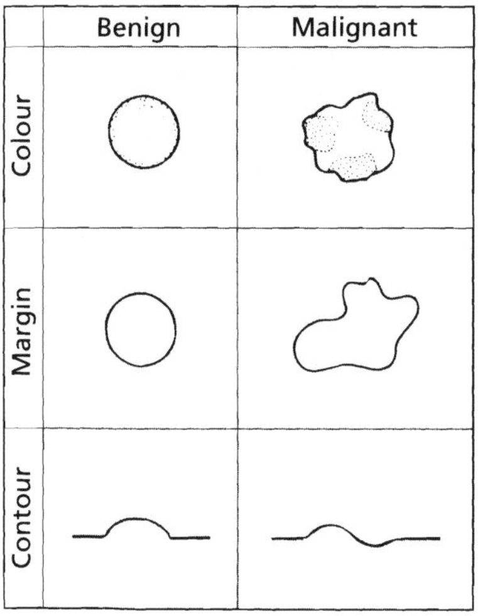

	Benign	Malignant
Colour	○	(irregular shape)
Margin	○	(irregular shape)
Contour	(smooth curve)	(irregular curve)

Fig. 2.1 Pigmented lesions. Benign pigmented tumours are usually uniform in colour and shape. Variation in colour, irregularity of margin and depth or ulceration suggests malignancy.

Plates 2.1–2.18 fall between pp. 28 and 29.

Table 2.1 Checklist for suspected malignant melanoma. From MacKie, R.M. (1990) Clinical recognition of early invasive malignant melanoma. *British Medical Journal* 301, 1005–1006.

Major signs	Minor signs
Change in size	Inflammation
Change in shape	Crusting or bleeding
Change in colour	Diameter >/=7 mm

A patient with a pigmented lesion showing any major sign should be considered for referral. The presence of additional minor signs are a further stimulus for referral.

papular, but retains the brown colour (compound naevus). Eventually the junctional component may be lost completely, and the tumour presents as a lightly pigmented or skin-coloured, fleshy papule (intradermal or cellular naevus). Benign naevi are often slightly hairy.

Seborrhoeic wart (seborrhoeic keratosis, basal cell papilloma) (Plate 2.2)
These warty, evenly pigmented, oval tumours with a 'stuck on' appearance are common in the elderly. They have no malignant potential.

Malignant melanoma (Plates 2.3–2.7)
The clinical features include:
• variation in colour: black/brown/blue/red/white areas. The tumour may be amelanotic;
• irregularity in margin;
• variation in depth;
• bleeding or ulceration;
• size greater than 7 mm.

Many tumours can mimic malignant melanoma. Patients with suspicious lesions should be referred to a specialist. The tumours must be completely excised and submitted for histology. Incisional biopsies probably do not increase the risk of metastasis but do make histological interpretation difficult because the overall architecture of the tumour cannot be assessed with an incomplete specimen.

Pyogenic granuloma (Plate 2.8)

This presents as a rapidly growing, exudative, vascular tumour often on a finger. The tumour can usually be differentiated from an amelanotic melanoma by the speed of growth.

Basal cell carcinoma (BCC, rodent ulcer)

Basal cell carcinomas are low-grade malignancies which are slow growing and locally invasive. They metastasize rarely. The common types are nodular, pigmented, superficial (multicentric) and morphoeic (sclerosing).

Nodular and pigmented BCC (Plate 2.9)

This is the commonest and most easily recognized variety of BCC. The tumour is rather translucent or 'pearly' and may have scattered telangiectasiae over the surface. It frequently ulcerates but retains the characteristic pearly rolled margin.

The pigmented nodular variety of BCC is occasionally mistaken for a malignant melanoma, but it is usually possible to demonstrate characteristic pearly areas within the tumour.

Superficial BCC (Plate 2.10)

There may be one or several flat, erythematous, crusted or scaly lesions, which are easily confused with eczema, psoriasis or Bowen's disease. Careful inspection of the lesion when the skin is stretched gently will reveal a raised pearly border.

Morphoeic BCC (Plate 2.11)

This type of BCC has an ill-defined margin and presents as an indurated, yellowish plaque, frequently with some telangiectasiae on the surface.

Kerato-acanthoma (Plate 2.12)

These benign tumours may cause alarm but the history of a rapid increase in size combined with the classical appearance, a cup-shaped nodule containing a central keratin plug, suggests the diagnosis of kerato-acanthoma. The pathologist will be

13

unable to confirm this diagnosis on a fragmented biopsy, so it is essential to excise or take an elliptical biopsy from one edge extending into the normal skin on the opposite side. The rest of the tumour can be curetted.

Solar keratosis (actinic keratosis) (Plate 2.13)
Small hyperkeratotic, brownish papules develop on sun-exposed skin, e.g. hands, forearms or scalp. These are premalignant lesions but some do regress spontaneously. In others an area of induration or ulceration may develop indicating the presence of a squamous cell carcinoma (SCC).

Bowen's disease (intra-epidermal SCC) (Plate 2.14)
Any erythematous, scaly, poorly-marginated lesion, which resembles eczema or psoriasis but which has not responded to treatment, should be biopsied to exclude Bowen's disease. A superficial BCC has a similar appearance but there is usually a slightly raised, pearly border which is more obvious if the skin is stretched. Long-standing Bowen's disease may eventually develop areas of induration and ulceration where frankly invasive SCC has supervened.

Squamous cell carcinoma (SCC) (Plates 2.15, 2.16)
This may develop *de novo* or where there has been a previous lesion, e.g. solar keratosis, radiotherapy necrosis, persistent varicose ulcer. Any solar keratosis which has areas of induration should be biopsied or excised. A SCC arising within a solar keratosis is usually well differentiated and the risk of metastasis is low; lesions on the lip and ear behave aggressively.

Dermatofibroma (histiocytoma; sclerosing haemangioma) (Plate 2.17)
These firm nodules, 0.5–3 cm in diameter, usually develop on the upper arm or leg, possibly as a reaction to insect bites or minor trauma. The tumours may be pigmented and the overlying epidermis can be smooth or rather warty. The firm consistency of the tumour suggests the diagnosis. The tumours

are benign and removal is not necessary. Excision may leave an unsightly scar, particularly on the arm.

Chondrodermatitis nodularis chronica helicis
(Plate 2.18)
Typically these tender lesions present on the rim of the ears of middle-aged or elderly men. The patient is unable to lie on the affected side because pressure causes pain. The small nodule may be ulcerated. Some patients have more than one lesion. Frequently chondrodermatitis nodularis is misdiagnosed as a skin cancer, but pain is not a feature of skin cancer. (See Chapter 8 for further information about treatment.)

Patient Preparation

A moment or two spent making sure that both patient and operator are comfortable will make all the difference to the smooth running of the procedure to be carried out. Make sure that all necessary equipment is in working order and close at hand. A good light is essential (Fig. 3.1a).

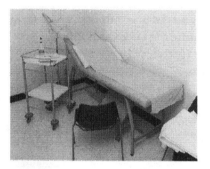

Fig. 3.1 (a) Layout of operating area.

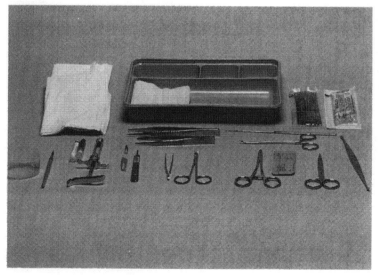

Fig. 3.1 (b) Layout of suggested instruments.

Positioning the patient

The patient should be lying down, however small the procedure. (The toughest looking person may feel dizzy at the sight of a needle, let alone an array of instruments!)

• *Head and neck procedures*. Raise the head of the patient and lower the legs. This will help to reduce the bleeding.

• *Hand procedures*. Place the oustretched hand on a table attached to the operating table or a trolley which can be positioned close to it.

The anxious patient

Simple explanation and reassurance is usually all that is necessary for these procedures.

Skin preparation

The affected area should be washed with a quick-acting alcoholic antiseptic such as 0.5% chlorhexidine in 70% alcohol (Hibisol). A non-alcoholic antiseptic should be used on the face or if using cautery.

Local anaesthesia

Agents

One per cent or 2% lignocaine with or without adrenaline; 1 in 200 000 is all that is necessary. Various agents are available with similar effect.

Toxicity

For the small lesions under discussion in this book, problems of toxicity will not arise. However, a guide to the maximum safe dose of lignocaine is as follows.

• 500 mg of lignocaine with adrenaline, i.e. 50 ml of 1% solution.

• 200 mg of lignocaine without adrenaline, i.e. 20 ml of 1% solution.

These levels are approximate and relate to normal adults. Preparations with adrenaline must not be used in any digital anaesthesia. It is safe to use adrenaline in the face, including the tip of the nose.

Syringes and needles

Ordinary disposable syringes using fine-gauge needles are adequate. The re-usable dental syringe with a cartridge and a very slender needle is preferable.

Technique

Local infiltration (Fig. 3.2)

1 Raise an intradermal bleb and continue injecting intradermally as the needle is slowly advanced.

2 Reinsert the needle in an area already infiltrated.

3 If undermining is necessary, ensure that a wide area is infiltrated at fascial level.

4 The scalp is highly vascular and the use of lignocaine with adrenaline is most suitable. The solution should be infiltrated both subcutaneously and beneath the galea aponeurotica for haemostatic and anaesthetic effect.

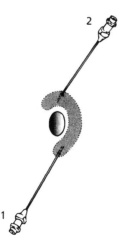

Fig. 3.2 Local infiltration. 1= first insertion of needle; 2=second insertion of needle into already anaesthetized skin.

Practical tips for children
It is possible to carry out some simple procedures in children. The topical local anaesthetic, 'EMLA' cream (Astra), when applied thickly under occlusion, e.g. with a 'tegaderm' patch for 2 h, will provide some skin anaesthesia. This can be supplemented with an injection of lignocaine which, if warmed and in a more dilute form than for adults, is less painful when injected.

Ring block (Fig. 3.3)
Adrenaline must never be used, 3–4 ml lignocaine is adequate.
1 One per cent or 2% plain lignocaine is used to raise an intradermal bleb on the dorsum of the finger to one side.
2 By palpating the volar surface, the tip of the needle is passed volarwards next to the bone in order to infiltrate the ipsilateral digital nerve.
3 The needle is then partially withdrawn and infiltration is continued across the dorsum of the finger.
4 The needle is then reintroduced through anaesthetized skin on the other side of the dorsum of the finger and again passed volarwards next to the bone in order to block the other digital nerve.
The same technique can be applied to the toes.

Tourniquets
These are essential when excising lesions or taking biopsies from the fingers.

Arm or leg
Exsanguinate the arm or leg either by using an Esmarch or Martin's bandage or by simple elevation of the limb for a couple of minutes.

A tourniquet at 250 mmHg for the arm and 400 mmHg for the leg will be tolerated by most patients for 5–10 min without anaesthesia.

If a proper tourniquet is unavailable, a sphygmomanometer can be used as a substitute (Fig. 3.4).

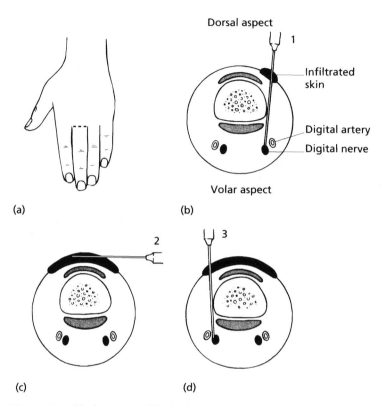

Fig. 3.3 Ring block. (a) Site of block. (b), (c), (d) Successive positioning of needle.

Fingers

Rubber tubing technique (Fig. 3.5)

The fine rubber tubing is fastened with mosquito forceps and tightened by twisting. It is vital to remember to remove it at the end of the procedure!

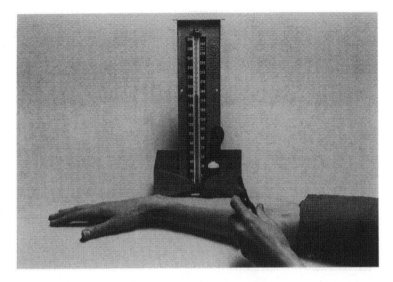

Fig. 3.4 Use of a sphygmomanometer as a tourniquet.

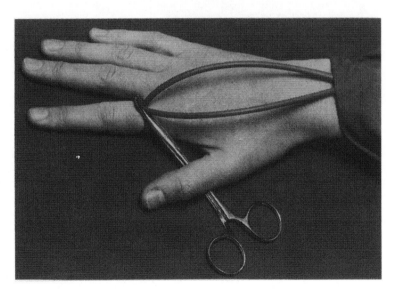

Fig. 3.5 Finger tourniquet using rubber tubing.

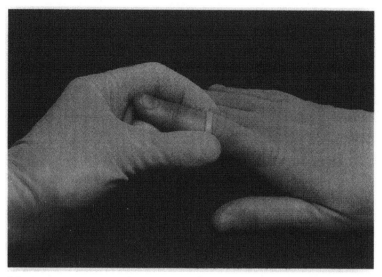

(a)

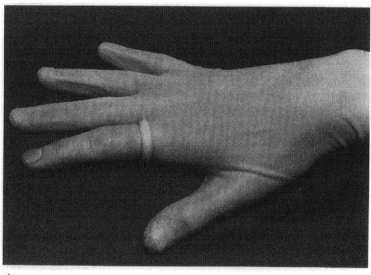

(b)

Fig. 3.6 (a) and (b) Finger tourniquet using glove technique.

Glove technique (Fig. 3.6)
This is a simple method which exsanguinates the finger, applies a tourniquet and covers the rest of the hand with something sterile.

A suitably sized surgeon's glove is put on the patient's washed hand. The rubber of the tip of the finger to be operated on is cut across and the glove is rolled down that finger.

Biopsy Techniques

Introduction
A good skin biopsy can provide valuable information, but a biopsy that is too small or too superficial, or one that is taken from a lesion that is atypical, too old, too young or excoriated may be useless.

It is essential to provide the pathologist with all the relevant clinical information, e.g. age of patient, history of lesion or rash, site of biopsy and previous treatment. A histological diagnosis provided without the clinical information may be misleading.

Non-specialists find it particularly difficult to diagnose inflammatory skin conditions and generally it is inappropriate for GPs to take biopsies from 'rashes' because they will have difficulty in correlating clinical and histological findings.

This chapter describes the methods of taking the skin biopsy and the indications for and limitations of each technique.

Shave biopsy

Indications
• Benign superficial epidermal lesions, e.g. seborrhoeic warts, solar keratoses.
• Benign intradermal naevi may be partially removed, but hyperpigmentation may recur and hairs nearly always regrow.

Disadvantage
Deep dermis and fat are not sampled.

Technique
1 The skin is cleaned.
2 Local anaesthetic is injected beneath the lesion to elevate it and facilitate removal.
3 A thin section is removed using a large scalpel blade (No. 22) held parallel to the skin. The surface should remain slightly raised. If nodules are shaved down to skin level, they heal with

a depressed scar, which may be more unsightly than the original lesion.

4 Haemostasis is obtained using pressure, a topical haemostatic agent (see Chapter 6) or gentle cautery.

Punch biopsy

The punch is a cylindrical cutting instrument which is available in varying diameters. A 4 mm punch provides an adequate tissue sample for histological examination.

Indications

1 To obtain a tissue sample from a tumour before definitive treatment.

2 To remove small lesions.

3 To provide small amounts of tissue for direct immunofluorescence, electron microscopy or culture.

4 To examine hair follicles; the punch must be orientated in the direction of hair growth and inserted deeply (Fig. 4.1).

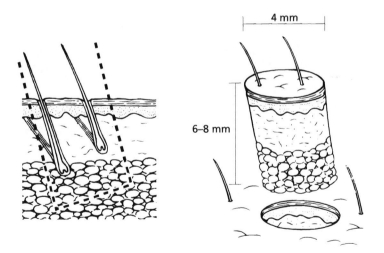

Fig. 4.1 Punch biopsy of the scalp: the angle of the biopsy must be orientated in the direction of hair growth and should extend into subcutaneous fat to avoid cutting off the more deeply situated follicles. Several deep 3–4 mm punch biopsies are generally more informative than a single elliptical specimen.

Disadvantages

This method of biopsy is rapid but there are limitations.

1 The sample is small and may not be representative of the whole lesion. An elliptical biopsy through a tumour demonstrates the architecture more clearly.

2 A punch biopsy does not show the transition from normal to abnormal skin.

3 Fat frequently sheers off. A punch biopsy is unsuitable for sampling lesions primarily in subcutaneous tissue, e.g. erythema nodosum.

4 In inexperienced hands, the complete anatomy of the hair follicle may not be demonstrated (see Fig. 4.1) and therefore an elliptical biopsy may be more satisfactory.

5 It may be difficult to orientate a small punch biopsy after fixation, so some pathologists prefer an elliptical specimen.

Technique

1 The skin is cleaned and anaesthetized.

2 The skin is held stretched at 90° to the natural wrinkle lines while the punch is inserted, pushed downward and twisted back and forth (Fig. 4.2). A slight 'give' is felt as the punch goes through the dermis. It is important to push the punch deep enough to obtain some underlying fat and provide an adequate tissue sample.

3 The punch is withdrawn. The core of tissue may come out with the punch. If it does not, the base can be cut with a pair of scissors or scalpel blade, while the surrounding skin is depressed to prevent blood obscuring the field. It may be necessary to lift up the specimen to separate it deeply.

4 The specimen should be gently removed with forceps or the scissors.

5 The circular defect will relax into an ellipse (see Fig. 4.2). Firm pressure will soon stop any bleeding. Generally sutures are not needed.

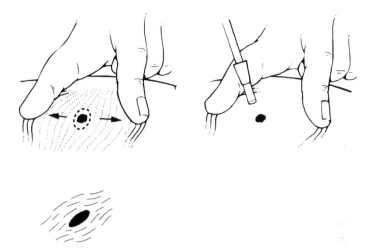

Fig. 4.2 Punch biopsy. If the skin is stretched perpendicular to Langer's lines, the circular defect relaxes into an ellipse which is easy to close with Steri-strips or a suture.

Elliptical biopsy

The biopsy may be *incisional* or *excisional*.

Indications

1 To examine the transition from normal to abnormal skin.

2 To examine the overall architecture of a lesion, e.g. kerato-acanthoma: a biopsy should always be taken right across the tumour, bisecting it.

3 To obtain samples from subcutaneous tissue, e.g. erythema nodosum, nodular vasculitis.

4 To obtain additional tissue for culture, direct immunofluorescence or electron microscopy. A single elliptical biopsy may be preferable to several small punch biopsies.

Incisional biopsy technique

1 The biopsy should extend from normal skin into the centre of the lesion, run parallel to the wrinkle lines and measure at least 1 cm in length.

2 The incision lines are marked with gentian violet or Bonney's blue.

3 The skin is cleaned and anaesthetized.

4 The skin is incised vertically down to subcutaneous tissues using a No. 15 scalpel blade. A second incision is made almost parallel to the first, meeting it at the corners, forming a narrow ellipse. The incisions must be vertical. If the wound edge is sloped there is less subcutaneous tissue removed, the specimen is unsatisfactory and the wound is more difficult to close (Fig. 4.3).

5 The specimen is lifted up gently by one corner. The base is cut with a scalpel as it is peeled back.

6 The wound is closed with interrupted sutures.

Elliptical excision technique
See Chapter 5.

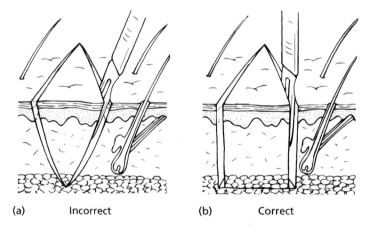

| (a) | Incorrect | (b) | Correct |

Fig. 4.3 Elliptical biopsy. (a) Incorrect. If the incisions are sloped, the biopsy does not contain adequate deep dermal or subcutaneous tissue and the wound is difficult to close. (b) Correct. The incisions are vertical, the specimen has plenty of deep dermis with some fat and the wound closes easily. If the pathology is mainly subcutaneous, e.g. erythema nodosum, the biopsy must extend deeply into the subcutaneous tissue.

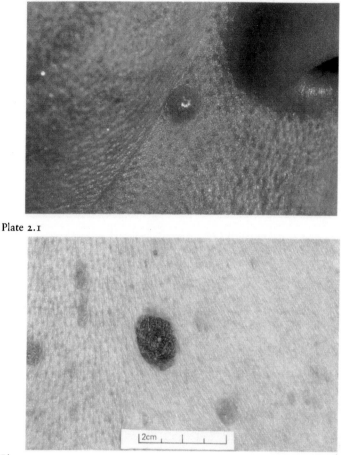

Plate 2.1

Plate 2.2

Plate 2.1 Acquired melanocytic naevus. The small dome-shaped papule has little residual pigment and a telangiectatic surface. It could be mistaken for a basal cell carcinoma, but the lesion had been present since childhood and was not changing.

Plate 2.2 Seborrhoeic wart (basal cell papilloma). This pigmented lesion has a well-defined, even outline and a warty surface, studded with small pits. The symmetry and the 'stuck on' appearance are characteristic. Paler, flatter seborrhoeic warts are also illustrated.

[facing page 28]

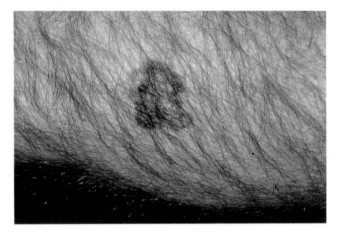

Plate 2.3

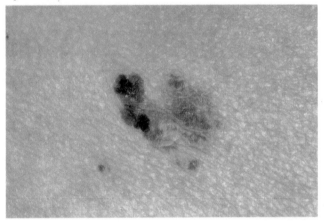

Plate 2.4

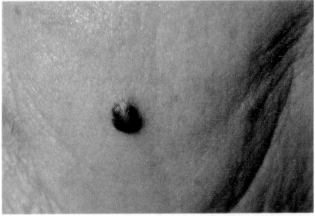

Plate 2.5

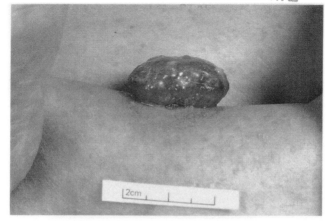

Plate 2.6

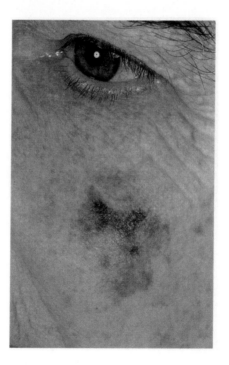

Plate 2.7

Plates 2.3–2.7 Malignant melanoma. The size, variation in colour and irregularity in outline suggest the diagnosis of malignant melanoma in these lesions (Plates 2.3, 2.4). Nodular melanomas are less asymmetrical, but in any pigmented lesion a history of change is worrying (Plate 2.5). Amelanotic melanomas may be more difficult to recognize, but this patient gave a clear history of a pre-existing pigmented lesion; a trace of pigment is present at the base of the tumour (Plate 2.6). A slow-growing irregularly pigmented lesion on the sun-exposed skin of an elderly patient is typical of *in situ* melanoma (lentigo maligna; Hutchinson's freckle) (Plate 2.7).

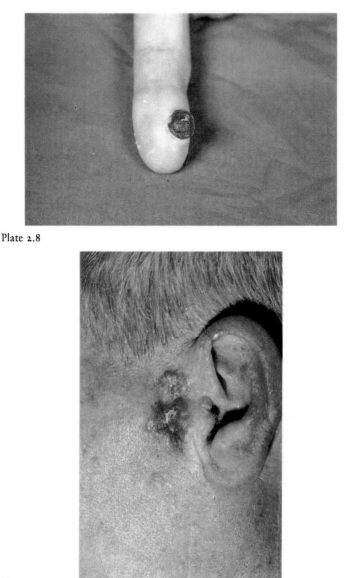

Plate 2.8

Plate 2.9

Plate 2.8 Pyogenic granuloma. This vascular tumour had grown rapidly over one or two weeks. Always consider the possibility of amelanotic malignant melanoma and ask the patient if there was a pre-existing pigmented lesion.

Plate 2.9 Nodular basal cell carcinoma (BCC). The pearly appearance, rolled edge and central ulcer are typical of a 'rodent ulcer'. Some areas in this BCC are pigmented. Tumours around the ear and nose may be deeply invasive.

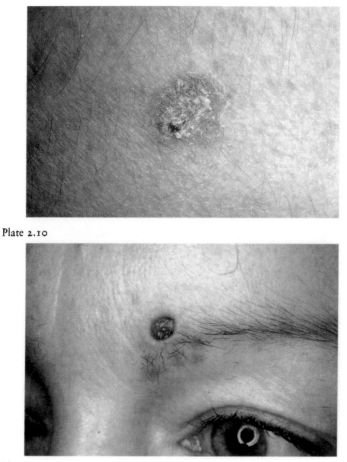

Plate 2.10

Plate 2.11

Plate 2.10 Superficial BCC. The slow-growing, scaly plaque mimics eczema, psoriasis or fungal infection; but topical treatments are ineffective. The raised border is easier to detect if the skin is stretched gently and lit from the side. This differentiates a superficial BCC from Bowen's disease.

Plate 2.11 Morphoeic BCC. The ill-defined, yellowish sclerosing plaque has ulcerated in this young woman.

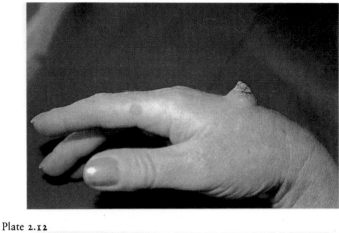

Plate 2.12

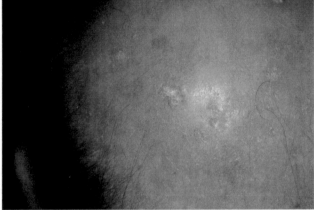

Plate 2.13

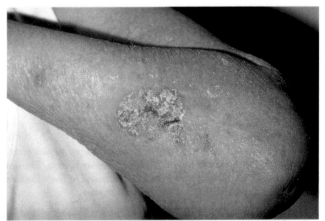

Plate 2.14

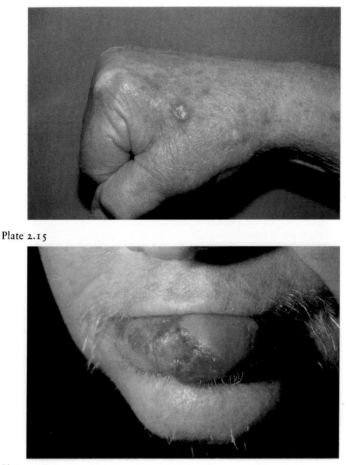

Plate 2.15

Plate 2.16

Plate 2.12 Kerato-acanthoma. The patient had a three-week history of a rapidly growing tumour. The rolled edge and central keratotic plug are characteristic of a kerato-acanthoma.

Plate 2.13 Solar keratosis. The bald scalp of this elderly man is extensively sun-damaged with pigmentation and many small keratoses.

Plate 2.14 Bowen's disease. An ill-defined slow-growing scaly plaque on the arm of an elderly patient. Bowen's disease, like a superficial BCC, is often misdiagnosed as eczema, psoriasis or a fungal infection.

Plates 2.15, 2.16 Squamous cell carcinoma (SCC). The risk of metastasis is low in this small, well-defined, indurated keratotic tumour (Plate 2.15). Squamous cell carcinomas arising on the lip have a much greater chance of metastasizing (Plate 2.16).

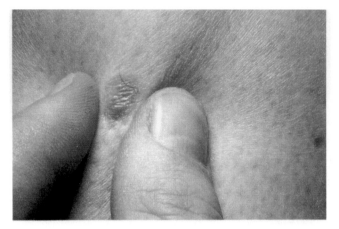

Plate 2.17

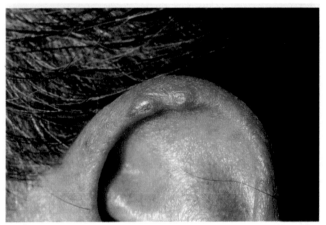

Plate 2.18

Plate 2.17 Dermatofibroma. The firm consistency of this reddish-brown tumour suggests the diagnosis. The tumour sinks into the dermis when the surrounding skin is compressed.

Plate 2.18 Chondrodermatitis nodularis chronica helicis. This man presented with two exquisitely tender nodules on his ear. These were keeping him awake. Both have developed small central ulcers. The history and appearance are typical of chondrodermatitis nodularis.

Practical points

1 Remember to photograph any unusual lesion before removing it.

2 Plan the investigations, obtain fixatives and culture mediums and if necessary talk to the pathologist so that you know how much tissue you need.

3 Choose the lesion.

(a) In most disorders, biopsy a fully developed lesion that is not scratched or secondarily infected.

(b) The edge is often the most active part of the lesion, e.g. annular erythemas.

(c) Bullous disorders: biopsy a fresh bulla less than 24 h old, or a pre-bullous urticarial lesion. The histology of older re-epithelializing bullae may be confusing.

(d) Direct immunofluorescence of bullous disorders: obtain perilesional skin. Direct immunofluorescence may be negative beneath the bulla. In dermatitis herpetiformis, normal skin from any part of the body is suitable for direct immuno-fluorescence examination.

(e) Vasculitis: biopsy lesions above the knee. The vasculature of the lower leg is already abnormal, damaged by venous hypertension and stasis.

4 Local anaesthetic.

(a) Inject it just under the skin to prevent the fluid in the skin distorting the anatomy.

(b) Lignocaine with adrenaline will cause mast cells to degranulate. In suspected urticaria pigmentosa, plain lignocaine should be injected around the biopsy site, not directly into it.

5 Special situations.

(a) *Kerato-acanthoma*: take a deep elliptical biopsy across the lesion including normal skin, the shoulder and the centre of the tumour.

(b) *Basal cell carcinoma*: never do a punch biopsy if you are planning to treat by curettage (see Chapter 6).

(c) *Malignant melanoma*: excise rather than incise any lesion suspected of being a malignant melanoma to obtain an accurate histological diagnosis.

(d) *Parapsoriasis versus mycosis fungoides*: take at least three biopsies, as foci of abnormal lymphocytes diagnostic of mycosis fungoides may be sparse. Monoclonal antibody studies may be used to define the T lymphocyte population.

Nail biopsy

The nail may be damaged by trauma, tumours or conditions such as psoriasis and lichen planus. Patients with an acquired nail dystrophy which cannot be explained should be referred to a specialist unit.

Details of the techniques used for nail biopsy are provided in: Baran, J. & Dawber, R. (1994) Nail Surgery and Traumatic Abnormalities. In: *Diseases of the Nails and their Management*, 2nd edn, pp. 345–415. Blackwell Science, Oxford.

Excision and Direct Closure

The maximum size of any lesion which can be excised and sutured directly is dependent on the mobility of the local skin.

Advantages of excision
1 The whole specimen can be submitted for histological diagnosis and completeness of excision.
2 Only one treatment is necessary.
3 Primary wound healing is usually achieved, giving a good cosmetic result.

Disadvantages
1 Local anaesthetic is required.
2 Aseptic technique, using sterilized surgical instruments, swabs and towels, is necessary.
3 A little time and a certain amount of operator skill are required.

Special areas
Special excision and reconstructive techniques may be required around the mouth and eyes to prevent distortion and ectropion, etc.

Patients with lesions in these areas should be referred to a specialist.

Some basal cell carcinomas of the inner canthal area, nasolabial area and around the ear tend to invade deeply and require more extensive excision with more complicated reconstruction. These patients should also be referred to a specialist.

Surgical technique

Marking the incision
Margins of excision should be marked prior to infiltration with local anaesthetic as this distorts the tissues.

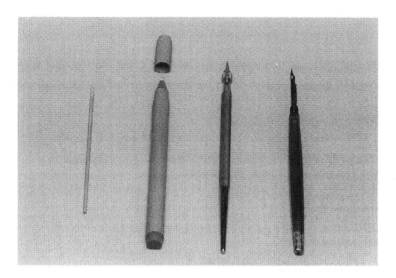

Fig. 5.1 Marking instruments. From left to right; wooden stick, sterile disposable fine fibre-tip pen, 'summerlad' pen, ordinary ink pen.

Marking instruments (Fig. 5.1)
Any of the following are suitable: tip of any fine instrument dipped in ink; sterile disposable fine fibre-tip pen or sterile pen and ink (Bonney's blue).

Approximate margins of excision
1 Benign lesions, 1–2 mm
2 Basal cell carcinomas (BCCs)
  nodular, 2–3 mm
  sclerosing, 6–8 mm
  multifocal, 8–10 mm
3 Bowen's, 3–4 mm
4 Squamous cell carcinomas (SCCs), 10–15 mm

Direction of ellipse
The shape of the lesion may suggest the direction of the ellipse but, if possible, the longitudinal axis of the ellipse should lie in or parallel to a natural skin crease.

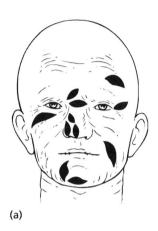

(a)

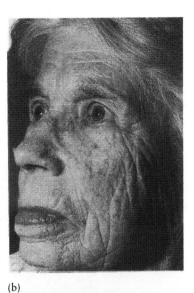

(b)

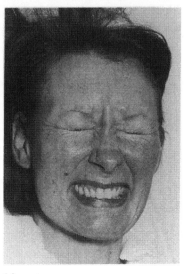

(c)

Fig. 5.2 (a) Suggested excision lines. (b) Old face showing natural skin creases. (c) Young face demonstrating skin creases.

1 *The face* (Fig. 5.2). In an older patient, the natural crease lines are easily visible (Fig. 5.2b). In the younger patient, these can be accentuated by asking the patient to smile, frown, raise eyebrows, close eyes tightly, purse lips, etc (Fig. 5.2c).

2 *The limbs.* Flexor aspects of joints do best with transverse incisions. Lesions over the extensor surfaces of joints may also be excised in a horizontal or oblique fashion if small enough. Pinch the skin with the joint fully flexed to determine the best direction for the excision. Longitudinal incisions are best for the rest of the limb.

3 *The trunk.* Langer's lines (Fig. 5.3) will act as guidelines for wound direction. If unsure about which direction is best, excise the lesion as a circle with skin under tension and note that the circle will tend to form an elliptical shape when the skin is relaxed (see Fig. 5.2a).

Dog ears and scar length

Any lesion excised as an ellipse will produce a scar of longer length than the original lesion. The main purpose of excising lesions as an ellipse is to reduce the formation of the dog ear. Small dog ears will settle in time and will be cosmetically acceptable. It may be difficult, at the time of marking, to assess

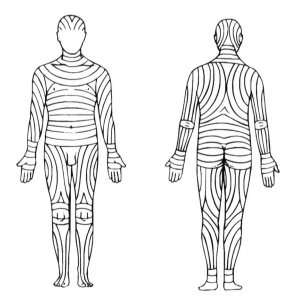

Fig. 5.3 Langer's lines.

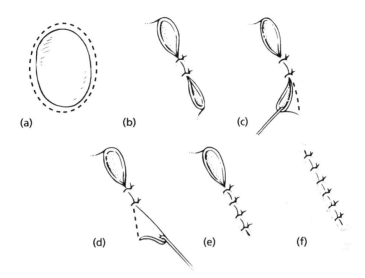

Fig. 5.4 (a) to (f) Sequence of excising dog ear subsequent to initial suturing.

how long the ellipse should be. The dog ear can always be excised subsequent to initial suturing (Fig. 5.4).

Atraumatic technique (Fig. 5.5)
Crushing tissue leads to devitalization of tissue which inevitably leads to poor healing and thus poor scars.

Skin edges should be handled with care. They should never be crushed by holding with any forceps, toothed or non-toothed. Fine-toothed forceps should be used to grip the dermis or to stabilize the skin edge with pressure. A skin hook could be used instead.

Knifecraft (Fig. 5.6)
A No. 15 blade is useful for almost any simple excision. Lax skin should be held under tension as the cut is made.

All incisions should be made vertical to the skin except in hair-bearing areas where it is advisable to angle the knife in the direction of the hair follicles in order to minimize damage to the follicles which might produce a bald patch.

35

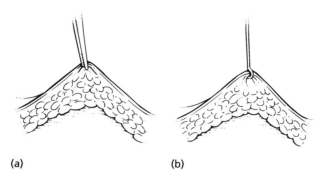

(a)   (b)

Fig. 5.5 Atraumatic technique. (a) Use of toothed forceps. (b) Use of skin hook.

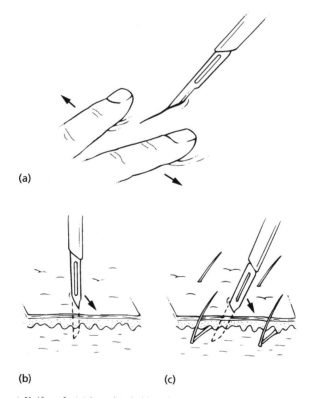

(a)

(b)   (c)

Fig. 5.6 Knifecraft. (a) Lax skin held under tension. (b) Incision vertical to skin. (c) Incision parallel to hair follicles in hair-bearing areas.

Undermining (Fig. 5.7)

Extent

Three to four mm of undermining should be carried out in all cases of excision in order to allow eversion of the wound edges when suturing. More undermining may be needed to take the tension off the wound edges.

Level

1 *Face* (Fig. 5.7a). The level of undermining should be just deep to the dermis in order to prevent damage to the facial nerve.

2 *Trunk and limbs* (Fig. 5.7b). Undermining is best carried out between superficial and deep fascia.

3 *Scalp* (Fig. 5.7c). Undermining should be carried out in the loose layer of areolar tissue between galea and pericranium. Multiple relaxation incisions on the deep surface of the galea may allow more advancement of the skin.

Danger. Undermining will always produce more bleeding and increase the risk of haematoma. After undermining more than a few millimetres, a few deep buried dermal sutures are advised to reduce the dead space and thus reduce the risk of haematoma (see p. 40).

Haemostasis

All bleeding can be stopped by applying pressure and waiting for a few minutes.

Various methods are available to speed up the haemostatic process.

1 Pressure.
2 Elevation of the limb.
3 Clipping vessels with mosquito forceps.
4 Tying vessels with 3/0 or 4/0 plain catgut.
5 Bipolar diathermy.
6 Mattress sutures in the scalp.

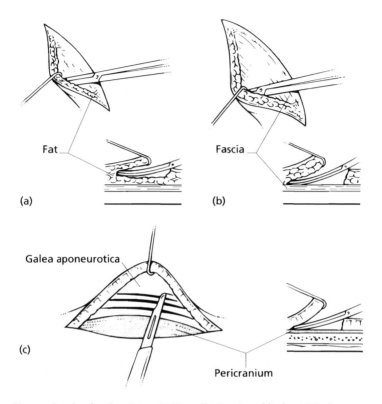

Fig. 5.7 Levels of undermining. (a) Face. (b) Trunk and limbs. (c) Scalp; multiple relaxation incisions.

Needlecraft
Table 5.1 gives details of suture materials and methods.

Suturing technique
The aim of suturing is to produce accurately apposed, everted wound edges in an atraumatic manner. This should produce healing by primary intention leading to a scar of good quality (see Chapter 9).

Always use tapercut needle. Never use a round-bodied needle. The operator should be comfortable, with a good light source. If

Table 5.1 Suture materials and methods.

Area	Suture method	Suggested suture material	Timing of suture removal
Scalp	Interrupted /mattress	3/0 or 4/0 Ethilon or Prolene	7–10 days
Face and neck	Interrupted	5/0 or 6/0 Ethilon or Prolene	5 days maximum
	Buried dermal	5/0 or 6/0 Vicryl and Steri-strips	48h minimum
Limbs and trunk	Buried dermal with sub-cuticular	3/0 or 4/0 Vicryl or 3/0 or 4/0 Prolene or Steri-strips	3 weeks 3 weeks As long as possible
	Interrupted	3/0 or 4/0 Ethilon or Prolene	10–14 days

an assistant is available, the wound can be stretched lengthwise between two skin hooks. This helps to stabilize the skin and makes suturing easier (see Fig. 5.8a)

There are several methods of suturing wounds as follows.

Simple interrupted (Fig. 5.8)

1 The needle should be placed in the needle-holder one-third to a half of the way along the curve from the suture material.

2 In the opposite hand, a pair of forceps (e.g. toothed Adson's) should be used to grip the dermis or stabilize the skin edge by applying pressure.

3 The needle tip should be inserted at 90° to the skin and it should be angled so as to take a large 'bite' of the deeper part of the skin.

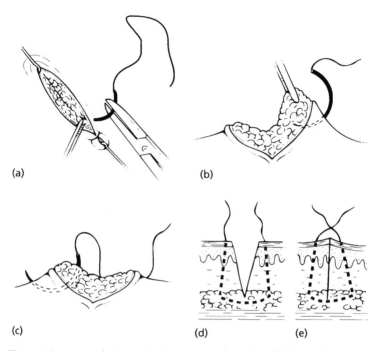

(a)

(b)

(c)

(d)

(e)

Fig. 5.8 Suturing technique—simple interrupted. (a) Use of skin hooks stabilizing the skin. (b) Insertion of needle at 90° to skin. (c) Equal 'bite' of opposing wound edge. (d), (e) Position and depth of suture.

4 An equal bite of skin must be taken from the outer edge of the wound and by lifting the skin edge with a hook or rolling the dermis outwards with a pair of toothed forceps, the deeper part of the bite will be wider and thus the skin edges will be everted. NB Inverted wound edges will produce depressed, ugly scars.

5 Tying knots using instruments allows more control over suture tension (Fig. 5.9). If the stitching is too tight, the wound edges will be strangulated and devitalized, leading to poor healing. If the stitching is too loose, the wound will gape. For a few days after the operation there will be some oedema in the wound edges and therefore stitches will apparently become tighter.

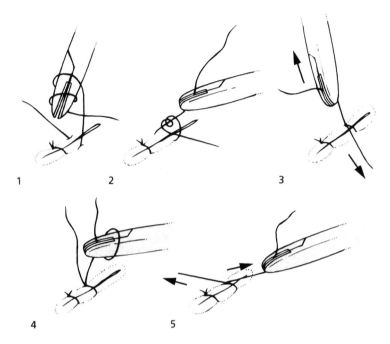

1   2   3

4   5

Fig. 5.9 Knot tying.

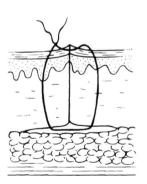

Fig. 5.10 Vertical mattress suture.

Vertical mattress (Fig. 5.10)

Use

1 In the scalp where it can be put in quite tightly to control the bleeding.

2 In other areas where the occasional mattress suture will help to evert the wound edges.

Technique

A simple interrupted suture is inserted taking good-sized 'bites' of the skin edges. The needle is then passed back across the wound superficially taking a much smaller but still everted bite.

Continuous subcuticular (Fig. 5.11)

Use

1 Where wound edges are straight and equal in length and depth.

2 Where wounds tend to stretch. This suture leaves no stitch marks and can therefore be left in for a longer time.

3 Where ease of suture removal is indicated, e.g. in young children.

Technique

1 With 3/o or 4/o nylon or Prolene, the needle is inserted about 1 cm away from one end of the wound and the end of the suture is held with a clip.

2 Equal bites are taken continuously along the length of the wound into the dermis only.

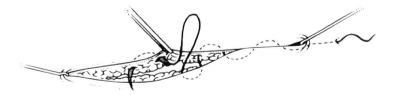

Fig. 5.11 Continuous subcuticular suture.

3 At the other end of the wound, the needle is brought out through the skin about 1 cm from the end.

4 The ends of the nylon or Prolene should be held down to the skin with Steri-strips.

5 With an absorbable suture such as Vicryl, the suture may be tied in a knot which is buried at each end of the wound.

6 These sutures may be left in for three or more weeks. They are usually easily removed by applying steady tension to one end of the nylon or Prolene. If the suture appears stuck, leave it for a few more weeks or attach an elastic band to one end and tape the elastic band to the skin and the suture will be slowly removed by steady tension.

Deep buried (Fig. 5. 12a)

This suture takes the tension off the skin edges and helps to close the dead space, thus reducing the likelihood of haematoma.

Use

1 In deeper wounds.

2 In undermined wounds.

3 If used with Steri-strips the suture should be modified to a buried dermal stitch (Fig. 5.12b).

Technique

With an absorbable 4/0 or 5/0 suture, the needle is inserted through the fat and includes a little dermis. The knot is buried deeply.

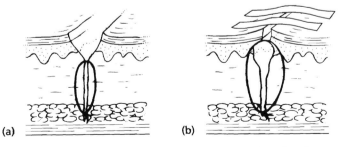

(a)   **(b)**

Fig. 5.12 (a) Deep buried suture. (b) Primary buried dermal stitch with Steri-strips.

Enucleation of cysts (Fig. 5.13)

Use
Epidermoid cysts, e.g. sebaceous cysts, pilar cysts, etc.

If the cyst has been previously infected, enucleation may be difficult and excision may be the treatment of choice.

Technique
1 A small elliptical incision is made around the punctum if present.
2 Using curved scissors or a scalpel, the cyst wall is dissected from the surrounding tissues and removed in one piece. If the cyst wall is breeched, the contents can be removed and the lining avulsed.

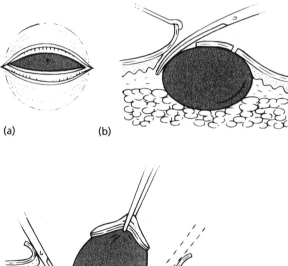

(a)   (b)

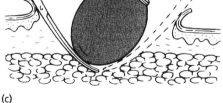

(c)

Fig. 5.13 Enucleation of cysts. (a) Elliptical incision around punctum. (b) and (c) Dissection around cyst.

3 The wound is closed in two layers to close the dead space left after the removal of the cysts.

NB *Infected sebaceous cysts* should be either curetted or left to settle and excised when quïescent.

Recurrent sebaceous cysts on the face are best excised under general anaesthesia and therefore should be referred to specialist units.

Wound dressings (Fig. 5.14)

Wounds form a coagulum naturally and quickly and therefore 'plastic' dressing sprays are really unnecessary and can make subsequent suture removal difficult.

1 *Scalp.* No dressing is required; the patient should be instructed not to wash his hair for a couple of days.

2 *Face.* Steri-strips can be used to take the tension off the wound edges. No other dressing is required. Again the wound should not be manipulated for a couple of days.

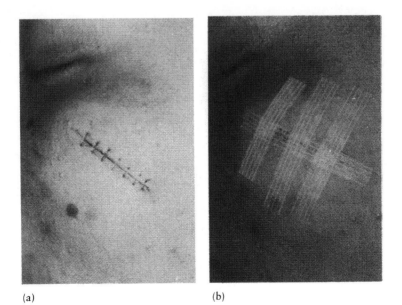

(a)   (b)

Fig. 5.14 (a) and (b) Wound dressing—use of Steri-strips.

3 *Trunk and limbs.* Steri-strips can be applied. A simple gauze dressing may be necessary for comfort to prevent rubbing of the wound with clothes, etc.

4 *Hands.* Small wounds are usually no problem. Patients should be encouraged to elevate hands but should also maintain a full range of movement of all upper limb joints.

5 *Legs.* Wounds heal better with rest and elevation. A supportive bandage (e.g. crêpe and/or Tubigrip) should be applied from toe to knee. The patient should be instructed to walk around or to sit with his feet up. He should not stand still for long periods or sit with his feet remaining dependant.

CHAPTER 6

Curettage, Cautery and Diathermy

This chapter describes some simple alternatives to excision and discusses the indications for their use.

Curettage

The classical curette is a spoon-shaped instrument available in various sizes. It is used to remove small, well-defined tumours on sites with a firm base and minimal mobile tissue, e.g. ears, nose, forehead. Soft abnormal tissue is easily scraped off but the curette has little effect on normal dermis (Fig. 6.1). Haemostasis is obtained with pressure, a topical agent (see below), cautery or diathermy. The ring curette, usually provided as a disposable instrument, is a sharper, more precise tool. The edge is so keen that minimal effort is required and this reduces shearing force. However greater experience is needed to avoid damaging normal tissue. It is less good when dealing with veruccae but gives better results for seborrhoeic warts on lax skin.

Indications

Superficial lesions

1 Molluscum contagiosum and filiform warts. These may be rapidly removed with a fine ring curette. Local anaesthetic is not always necessary.

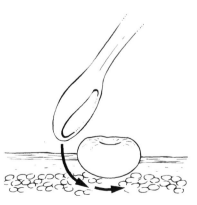

Fig. 6.1 Curettage: soft, abnormal tissue is easily distinguished from the firm normal dermis. Fibrosing or scarred tumours cannot be removed with a curette.

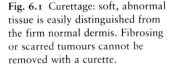

2 Seborrhoeic warts (seborrhoeic keratoses). The tumour is anaesthetized, the curette inserted at one edge and the lesion peeled off. Haemostasis is obtained with pressure or a topical agent. Curettage may be combined with cryosurgery. The tumour is frozen with liquid nitrogen until it just turns white. This anaesthetizes the area and the lightly frozen tumour can be peeled off using the curette. If the keratosis is frozen too deeply it will be difficult to remove.

3 Actinic (solar) keratoses, Bowen's disease. It is impossible to assess the presence or absence of invasion using curetted specimens. If there is any question of an underlying squamous cell carcinoma (SCC), a biopsy should be taken from the suspicious area immediately before curettage. The curette is used to remove abnormal epidermis and the base is lightly cauterized or electro-dessicated to prevent recurrence.

4 Solitary plantar warts (verruca). Recently acquired or spreading veruccae are unlikely to be cured by surgical treatment. However a well-defined, solitary plantar wart which has been present for two years will probably not recur if removed by curettage.

(a) The patient lies prone with the leg flexed at the knee so that the foot is elevated (Fig. 6.2).

(b) Lignocaine without adrenaline is injected around the wart. This is often very painful. It may be possible to start the injection in thinner skin on the side of the foot or heel and then to work towards the verucca by injecting through already anaesthetized skin.

(c) The foot is dorsiflexed and held with the operator's thumb pressed down firmly on the skin adjacent to, and just proximal to, the wart to reduce bleeding.

(d) The wart is scooped out with a curette while firm digital pressure is maintained.

(e) The base and edges are scraped to remove residual wart tissue. Any redundant skin around the edge of the wound can be trimmed with scissors.

(f) Light cautery or topical agents provide haemostasis.

(g) A firm dressing is applied.

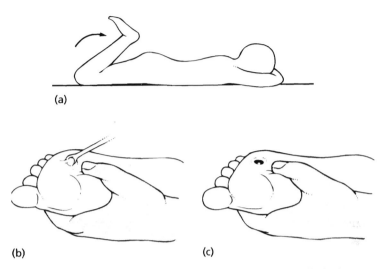

(a)

(b)   (c)

Fig. 6.2 Curettage of a plantar wart. (a) The patient is prone with the foot elevated. (b) The wart is anaesthetized and removed by curettage while the operator's thumb applies firm pressure to prevent blood obscuring the field. (c) A topical haemostatic agent is applied before digital pressure is released.

Postoperative care
These superficial wounds heal rapidly over in one to two weeks. They should be protected with dry dressings.

Nodular tumours
Excision and primary closure may be difficult. Curettage is a reasonable alternative to excision in selected cases.
1 Benign tumours, e.g. viral wart, kerato-acanthoma, pyogenic granuloma.
2 Malignant tumours, e.g. basal cell carcinoma (BCC). This is an area fraught with problems and curettage is unlikely to be an appropriate option in general practice. This method is used by some experienced practitioners especially for small tumours (≤ 5 mm in diameter) in individuals prone to multiple basal cell carcinomas. Generally, excision with appropriate margins and histological assessment of the adequacy of treatment is recommended.

Advantages
1 Simple, rapid technique.
2 No complicated equipment required.

Disadvantages
1 The wound heals slowly by secondary intention in three to six weeks. The hypopigmented scar may be hypertrophic, but improves with time. It is generally more noticeable than the linear scar obtained after excision and primary closure.
2 It is not possible to assess the presence or absence of dermal invasion in curetted fragments.
3 Fibrotic tumours cannot be removed.
4 Accurate curettage is impossible in the presence of scar tissue, e.g. from a previous biopsy.
5 Malignant tumours with ill-defined borders or in 'high risk' areas, e.g. nasolabial fold, medial canthus, cannot be completely removed by curettage. These tumours have deeper and wider extensions. The recurrence rate after curettage is unacceptably high.
6 Curettage on the scalp may cause an area of alopecia.

Technique
1 The tumour is cleaned and anaesthetized.
2 A preliminary deep biopsy is taken if indicated:
    (a) before removal of a kerato-acanthoma so that the pathologist can assess the architecture and depth of the tumour;
    (b) if there is any question of an underlying invasive SCC, e.g. an indurated actinic keratosis or indurated Bowen's disease.
3 A large curette is used to remove the tumour in one piece. The curette is inserted at one edge and the tumour scooped out.
4 The rim and base are thoroughly scraped with a small curette to remove any residual tumour.
5 Bleeding is controlled with a combination of pressure and a topical agent, cautery or electrodessication.
6 To ensure destruction of a BCC, a 2 mm rim of a surrounding normal tissue is cauterized. All the coagulated tissue is removed with the curette. Cautery and curettage of the whole area is

repeated two or three times. Vigorous use of cautery makes up for lack of skill with a curette, but increases scarring. Some dermatologists use the curette to define the overall shape of the BCC and follow this by excising a further 2 mm margin of normal skin. Interestingly, histological assessment of the curette margin shows residual tumour in 17% of cases.

Postoperative care

Curettage and cautery or curettage and electrodessication of nodular tumours leave an open wound which heals by secondary intention. The rate of healing depends on the amount of tissue destruction and the location of the tumour.

1 Daily dressings are required to absorb exudate. It may take one to three weeks for a crust to form.

2 Care must be taken to protect the wound from trauma and keep it dry. It heals in three to six weeks.

3 A rim of erythema usually develops around the healing wound. This does not imply infection.

4 Bleeding within the first three days may occur because of inadequate electrocoagulation. Bleeding may also be a complication when the eschar separates between days 10 and 14.

5 The risk of infection is low.

Topical haemostasis

Superficial haemostasis is required after shave biopsy or curettage. Pressure will eventually stop the bleeding, but the process can be accelerated without increasing the amount of tissue destruction, by using a topical protein precipitating agent.

Topical haemostatic agents

• Monsel's solution (basic ferric sulphate (67.5 g) dissolved in distilled water (95 ml) by boiling and stirring and after cooling made up to 100 ml with distilled water).

• Aluminium chloride hexahydrate can be made at 30–50% strengths. It is commercially available for the treatment of hyperhidrosis as Driclor (Stiefel) and Anhydrol Forte (Dermal).

• 30% to 50% aluminium chloride in 50% isoprophyl alcohol.

- 25% to 50% trichloracetic acid.
- 20% to 50% silver nitrate solution or silver nitrate sticks.

Monsel's solution and aluminium chloride solution are the agents of choice. They produce a superficial layer of coagulated tissue without increasing the size of the wound. Silver nitrate is widely used in Britain, but it causes unpredictable tissue destruction which delays wound healing and increases scarring. Trichloracetic acid is an excellent haemostatic agent but can damage the surounding skin and enlarge the wound.

Method of application
A gauze swab is used to dry the surface of the wound before the haemostatic agent is applied.

A cotton-tipped applicator is dipped into the haemostatic agent and immediately the swab is removed the applicator is pressed onto the wound with a rolling motion.

Electrocautery

The hot wire cautery employs a small voltage to generate a current which heats an element with a high resistance. The hot element, a wire loop or needle, is used to burn the tissues or coagulate small vessels. Temperature can be adjusted. No current passes through the body.

Indications
1 Removal of benign superficial pedunculated skin tumours that do not require biopsy, e.g. skin tags, condyloma acuminatum, pedunculated naevi.
2 Destruction of small benign vascular tumours.
3 Combined with curettage for the destruction of BCCs, pyogenic granulomas and kerato-acanthomas (see page 50).

Advantages
1 Simple rapid technique.
2 The heat sterilizes the instrument and the skin.
3 Bleeding is minimal.

Disadvantages

1 The smell of burnt flesh is unpleasant for the patient.
2 Healing is slow.
3 Scarring is unpredictable and may be hypertrophic, but improves with time.

Practical tip

Necrotic tissue delays healing and increases scarring. Cauterize lightly and use pressure to obtain haemostasis.

Diathermy (Fig.6.3)

In electrocautery, heat is induced in a wire loop by its resistance to an electric current. Diathermy derives from the Greek meaning 'through heat' but does not emphasize the important element, namely that an electric current passes through the tissues. Low frequency currents produce electrolysis and muscle contraction but little heat, whereas the main effect of high frequency currents is heating. Other variables which determine the type of tissue injury are the wave form, the duration of application and the size of the electrode. High voltage, small currents produce electrodessication while low voltage, large currents coagulate or even cut.

Electrodes and diathermy burn

The small active electrode produces a high current density and local heat. The current is dissipated through the tissues with the body acting as a capacitor. If no indifferent plate electrode is used, the body should be insulated. Otherwise current may pass to metallic parts of the table causing a burn at the point of contact. Low output monoterminal machines (e.g. Birtcher Hyfrecator) may be used in this way with minimal risk. It is good practice to use a plate electrode and this should be in good contact with the patient's skin and attached so that it will not become loose with movement of the patient.

Electrodessication

This is a rapid method of destroying small avascular benign

Indifferent plate electrode

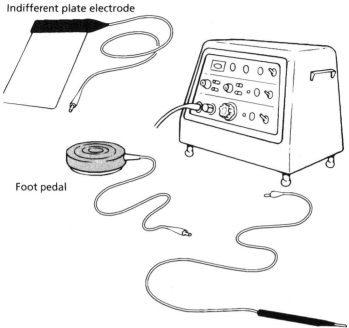

Foot pedal

Active electrode

Fig. 6.3 Diathermy machine.

lesions by dehydration. If the lesion is highly vascular the current is dissipated rapidly and the effect is reduced. The current is 'cool' so that the stoical patient may not need local anaesthetic. There is a risk of transferring infection, such as hepatitis B, by reusable electrodes. They should be properly sterilized or disposable electrodes used instead.

Indications
1 Multiple benign avascular lesions that do not require a biopsy, e.g. skin tags, filiform warts, seborrhoeic keratoses.
2 May be used in preference to topical haemostatics after curettage or shave excisions.

Advantages
1 A rapid method of destroying small lesions.
2 Minimal scarring, provided the power is kept low.

Disadvantages

1 May be painful, but multiple injections of local anaesthetic may be both unpleasant and impractical.

2 Cannot be used for vascular lesions as the current is dispersed by the blood and is less effective.

Technique

1 A monoterminal needle electrode is used.

2 The diathermy machine is adjusted to a low setting.

3 The electrode is inserted into the lesion.

4 A short pulse of current is released.

5 The tissue is 'dried out', turns white and small blood vessels are thrombosed. The destruction is superficial.

6 Blood disperses the current and reduces its effect. If the power is increased to compensate, the process is painful and more destructive electrocoagulation occurs (see below).

Postoperative care

The skin should be kept dry. The crust is shed after 10–14 days.

Electrocoagulation

Electrocoagulation is a more destructive process than electro-dessication. An intense heat is produced to char tissue. There is deep tissue destruction approximately equal to the visible lateral spread of charring.

1 Adequate coagulation for most dermatological procedures is produced using a monopolar electrodessicating needle electrode with a moderate output (see below).

2 More effective electrocoagulation is produced by combining an active electrode with an indifferent plate electrode. An active ball electrode is sometimes used to dissipate current over a large area, but as the current density is decreased the output must be increased and this causes deeper tissue destruction. The tissue frequently sticks to the electrode and pulls away as it is removed, so that bleeding starts again.

3 The active and indifferent electrodes may be combined in one

handle so that there is no need for the plate electrode and there is less tissue destruction.
(a) A rigid bipolar electrode. This is suitable for coagulating small skin lesions.
(b) Bipolar forceps. Bleeding vessels may be precisely located and coagulated with minimal tissue destruction.

Indications
1 Small vascular lesions (e.g. angiomas, spider telangiectases) which do not require a biopsy.
2 Following curettage of a BCC, coagulation may be used to induce further tissue destruction.
3 Combined with curettage, as an alternative to cautery, to treat some BCCs.

Advantages
A simple, rapid technique which may be repeated. Scarring is minimal if the coagulation is brief.

Disadvantages
Tissue destruction is more extensive than with electrodessication.

Technique (for spider angioma)
1 The skin is cleaned.
2 The lesion should be clearly marked since it may be difficult to identify after local anaesthetic is injected. The central feeding vessel of a spider telangiectasia should be identified by attempting to blanche the lesion with pinpoint pressure.
3 Local anaesthetic is injected when necessary.
4 A needle electrode is inserted into the centre of the lesion.
5 A moderate strength current is passed briefly into the lesion to produce blanching. The lesion should not be over-treated or an unsightly scar may be produced. Coagulation can always be repeated later.

Postoperative care
The skin should be kept dry. A crust will form. This is shed after about 10–14 days but the skin may remain slightly erythematous for about a month.

Practical tip
Record the diathermy setting used in the patient's records so that the treatment can be repeated or adjusted as required.

Cryosurgery

Cryosurgery (cryotherapy) is defined as the deliberate destruction of diseased tissue by cold in a controlled manner. Cryosurgery should only be used when a confident clinical diagnosis has been made.

Liquid nitrogen is the commonly used refrigerant and is applied using a cotton wool swab, cryospray gun (Fig. 7.1), or cryoprobe (Fig. 7.1b). It is stored in a vacuum container. Great care must be taken when handling liquid nitrogen to avoid splashing exposed skin.

Cell injury and death are dependent on the following factors.
1 The final temperature reached: a temperature of −40°C or lower is necessary to kill cells by freezing alone, but in the clinical situation other factors such as ischaemia, inflammation

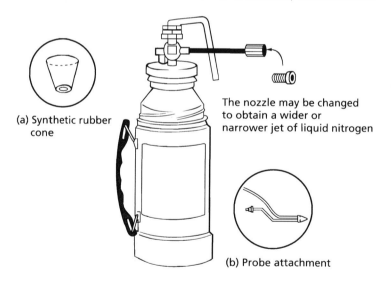

(a) Synthetic rubber cone

The nozzle may be changed to obtain a wider or narrower jet of liquid nitrogen

(b) Probe attachment

Fig. 7.1 Cryosurgery unit. A jet of liquid nitrogen is sprayed out of the nozzle. (a) Cone spray technique. Hollow cones are available in various sizes. The spray is directed into a fine cone which is placed over the lesion; surrounding structures are protected. The technique is particularly useful around the eye. (b) The probe attachment can be used instead of the nozzle if a deeper freeze is required. Pressure can be applied to the lesion while it is being frozen.

and an immunological response may assist in tissue destruction. A final temperature of $-25\,°C$ is probably adequate, certainly for benign lesions.

2 The rate of cooling: a rapid rate causes more tissue damage.

3 The thaw time: a prolonged thaw increases tissue damage.

Two freezes with a slow intervening thaw are more destructive than a single prolonged freeze. The greater the number of successive freeze–thaw cycles the greater the cell death—and morbidity.

Clinical effects

Pain

The patient usually feels a burning sensation during freezing and thawing. Local anaesthetic is not required for short freeze times but may be indicated when treating malignant tumours with double or multiple freeze–thaw cycles (see Further reading, p. 64). There is considerable individual variation in the pain threshold.

Freezing the forehead often produces a migraine-like pain and freezing plantar, palmar and periungual lesions may be particularly painful.

Postoperative pain is usually minimal.

Inflammation

Individuals vary enormously in their response to cryosurgery. Some oedema is common especially in areas where the skin is lax (e.g. periorbital). Blisters may form sometimes after minimal treatment, and are occasionally haemorrhagic.

Bleeding

Generally, this is not a problem.

Infection

Secondary infection is uncommon. Wounds remain moist with exudation of necrotic tissue for several weeks after a prolonged freeze. This is occasionally misinterpreted as infection.

Nerve damage
Local paraesthesiae or hypoaesthesia are not uncommon. Superficial nerves may be damaged by freezing leading to paraesthseiae or hypoaesthesia. The perineurium is unaffected and the nerve regrows along its sheath, so damage is usually temporary. However, care should be taken in areas where nerves are superficial, e.g. the elbow, sides of the fingers.

Pigment changes
A ring of perilesional postinflammatory hyperpigmentation is common. Hypopigmentation is frequently produced at the site of freezing and with prolonged freezes this may be permanent.

Cartilage
Cartilage is not usually damaged by the freeze times used in clinical practice. Therefore cryosurgery may be the treatment of choice for lesions on sites such as the ears and nose.

Wound healing
Dermal collagen is relatively resistant to damage by freezing. The lesions heal without wound contracture. The rate of healing depends on the depth of freeze, the site and the patient. After a short freeze, the wound usually forms a crust in a week.

Indications
1 Superficial keratotic lesions: seborrhoeic warts, viral warts, actinic keratoses, Bowen's disease.
2 Pigmented lesions: benign lentigines. The clinician *must* be sure the lesion is benign.
3 Malignant tumours: these should only be treated by experienced surgeons in specialist centres, using an aggressive spray technique. Long freeze–thaw cycles cause severe necrosis. Cryosurgery should not be used to treat tumours with ill-defined margins or those invading subcutaneous tissue. Cryosurgery does not normally cause cartilage necrosis and is particularly suitable for treating tumours on the ear. Suitable tumours may include:

(a) Superficial and nodular basal cell carcinomas (BCCs).

(b) Basal cell naevi (Gorlin's syndrome).

(c) Small, well-differentiated squamous cell carcinomas (SCCs) arising in actinic keratoses.

Contraindications

1 Children: most children under 7 years of age should not be expected to tolerate cryosurgery.

2 Pigmented skin: cryosurgery destroys melanocytes and even short freezes may cause permanent hypopigmentation. Cryosurgery should be avoided in patients with dark skin.

3 Legs: cryosurgery may not be the best mode of treatment for lesions below the knee because it may take several months for the wound to heal, particularly in elderly patients.

4 Periungual lesions: cryosurgery is very painful and may damage the nail matrix as well as the extensor tendon.

The swab technique

Advantages

A rapid, simple technique which requires no complicated apparatus. Sterility is not a problem.

Disadvantages

1 Cannot freeze widely or deeply as the swab rapidly rewarms and must be dipped repeatedly into the reservoir of liquid nitrogen.

2 Difficult to standardize, therefore this method is not suitable for malignant tumours.

3 Theoretically, viruses could be transferred to the flask if the same swab is used repeatedly.

Technique

A cotton wool swab is dipped into the reservoir of liquid nitrogen. The lesion is touched with the swab, applying pressure if a deep freeze is required.

The skin will turn white. Care is taken to avoid dripping

liquid nitrogen on to normal skin. A freeze time of between 5 and 15 s after visible ice formation is adequate for most superficial lesions see Table 7.1. Even 5 s may cause big blisters in some individuals, so always use a short freeze for the first treatment and record the freeze-time in the clinical notes.

Spray technique

Advantages
1 A rapid technique.
2 Haemostasis is complete.
3 No suturing is required.
4 Sterility is not a problem.
5 Multiple lesions may be treated.
6 Cartilage necrosis does not usually occur.
7 Scarring is minimal and the cosmetic result is excellent. Hypertrophic scarring occurs rarely.

Disadvantages
1 Immediate postoperative oedema.
2 Dressings required to absorb the exudate for 1–4 weeks after prolonged freezes.
3 Some patients suffer considerable discomfort during the treatment.
4 In pigmented or telangiectatic skin, the hypopigmentation is prominent and may be disfiguring.

Technique
1 A biopsy should be taken if the clinician cannot make a confident clinical diagnosis. In the rare instance that cryosurgery is indicated to treat a malignant lesion, the diagnosis must be confirmed histologically before treatment.
2 Local anaesthetic is not required for single freeze–thaw cycles (up to 30 s).
3 The aim is to produce an iceball which extends 2 mm onto normal skin. If the borders of the lesion are not clear, they should be marked prior to treatment.

Table 7.1 Freeze times for the treatment of benign and pre-malignant lesions. Standardization is difficult but whether using swab or spray technique the aim is to produce an iceball which extends 2 mm onto normal skin. Freeze times are measured after the formation of a solid iceball over the lesion or marked field.

Lesion	Practical tips and approximate freeze time
Actinic (solar) keratosis	5–10 s, or consider medical treatment in patients with widespread sun-damage (Chapter 8)
Bowen's disease	15–20 s, below the knee this will cause an ulcer and healing will be delayed. Medical treatment may be more appropriate (Chapter 8)
Seborrhoeic wart	10 s, alternatively seborrhoeic warts may be lightly frozen for 5 s and simply peeled off with a curette (NB freezing anaesthetizes the skin)
Solar (senile) lentigo	5–10 s, biopsy any flat pigmented lesion to establish the diagnosis before using cryosurgery
Molluscum contagiosum	10 s, molluscum do resolve spontaneously and are best ignored. 'Pox' scars are a common sequel. The lesions can be curetted after using a topical anaesthetic (EMLA cream) and this may be less painful than cryosurgery
VIRAL WARTS Common wart	10 s
Filiform wart	5–10 s, often best curetted
Plantar wart	Respond poorly to cryosurgery, which may be extremely painful. Always pare down to relieve pain. Once asymptomatic they are best ignored
Solitary plantar wart	15–30 s, consider curettage (Chapter 6)
Mosaic plantar wart	Double 30 s freeze–thaw cycle for the insistent stoic
Periungual wart	Cryosurgery is painful. Aggressive treatment may damage the nail matrix. These warts are particularly resistant to treatment
Genital warts	5–10 s, topical podophylline may be more appropriate Before treatment, adults should be referred to a department of genito-urinary medicine to be screened for other sexually transmitted diseases Children should be referred to a paediatrician for exclusion of sexual abuse

4 The spray tip is held close to the lesion. Small lesions are frozen by directing the spray at the centre of the lesion until the iceball encompasses the entire lesion. Larger (2–3 cm) superficial lesions may be treated using a 'paint–spray' technique: a steady jet of liquid nitrogen is moved back and forth across the surface until the entire lesion is frozen. A plastic teaspoon can be used to cover and protect the eye while treating periocular lesions.

5 Timing commences once solid ice has formed over the entire lesion (see Table 7.1).

6 The jet of liquid nitrogen is adjusted to maintain an iceball of a constant size.

7 Larger lesions and malignancies are more difficult to treat. The patient should be referred to a specialist (see Graham *et al.* (1992) for further information).

Postoperative care

1 Dressings are sometimes required to absorb excudate.

2 Tense blisters should be punctured with a clean needle.

3 A crust usually forms in one to two weeks. At this stage the lesion should be kept dry and protected from trauma.

4 The skin is initially erythematous, but this fades leaving a hypopigmented macule.

Further reading

Dawber, R., Colver, G. & Jackson, A. (1992) *Cutaneous Cryosurgery*. Martin Dunitz, London.

Special Techniques

Free skin grafts for leg ulcers

Leg ulceration is a common problem which is treated by a variety of specialists and GPs. The mainstay of treatment involves the management of the underlying cause and associated non-surgical dressing techniques. However, some ulcers benefit from a surgical approach which can range from a radical excision of the ulcer, along with identification and destruction of the perforating veins, to simple split skin grafting and small areas of pinch grafting. This section will describe the basic physiology of skin graft take and the use of pinch grafts. Radical excision of ulcers with split skin grafting is beyond the scope of this book and requires specialist surgical techniques. Preparation of leg ulcers prior to grafting, physiology of skin graft take and the technique of pinch grafting will be described.

Physiology of skin graft take

A skin graft may be partial thickness or full thickness. The graft is completely detached from the skin and placed on a vascular bed from which it derives its blood supply. The graft adheres to its new bed by the formation of fibrin. There is diffusion of nutrients through this fibrinous layer which keep the graft alive initially. Within two to three days, capillary linkage occurs with vascularization of the graft. The thinner the graft, the denser the capillary network in the superficial dermis and thus the easier the process of vascularization.

Sheering forces between graft and bed will prevent vascular link-up. Collection of haematoma or seroma between graft and bed will also prevent vascular link-up. The presence of haemolytic streptococci on the granulating surface almost invariably leads to graft failure.

Avascular recipient sites such as bare cortical bone, bare tendon and bare cartilage will not accept skin grafts. Skin grafts will only take on areas which can produce granulation tissue.

Preparation of ulcers prior to grafting

The appearance of healthy granulation tissue signals the right time to attempt skin grafting. 'Healthy' granulations are red, flat, free from slough and do not bleed readily. Marginal healing will be evident.

Local treatment of ulcers

There are a multitude of different topical preparations and types of dressings used in the management of leg ulcers. There are three main aims of local treatment prior to grafting.

1 Removal of dead tissue

This can be carried out by simply snipping away at any dead tissue in the ulcer as part of the daily dressing procedure. Some topical preparations (e.g. Flamazine, Aserbine, Furacin, etc.) help with the mechanical débridement by softening the eschar. Dead tissue is insensitive so that most débridement can be carried out without anaesthesia. Occasionally it may be necessary to débride the area under general anaesthesia.

2 Reduction of bacterial flora

Mechanical débridement and frequent changes of dressing will reduce the bacterial flora on all ulcers. Skin grafts will take even in the presence of some bacteria.

Haemolytic streptococci often give the granulations a glistening appearance and they must be eradicated before attempting skin grafting.

A heavy growth of *Pseudomonas pyocyanea* will make the dressings green and give off a characteristic odour. This organism is difficult to eradicate but its presence when granulations look healthy will not significantly reduce the amount of graft take. Phenoxyethanol 2.2% solution applied as a daily dressing will help to reduce the growth of pseudomonas.

Systemic antibiotics are only necessary for:
(a) eradication of haemolytic streptococci, or
(b) treatment of patients with cellulitis and systemic disturbance secondary to infected ulcers.

3 Maintenance of healthy granulations

Pale, oedematous granulations may be improved by using hypertonic saline dressings (2 × Normal). Alginates such as kaltostat or hydrocolloids such as Granuflex are useful in the maintenance of healthy granulation tissue and will aid healing along with sustained external pressure and elevation of the leg.

Anaesthesia

Most small ulcers can be grafted under local anaesthesia. Care must be taken not to exceed the maximum safe dose of lignocaine when infiltrating large areas of both recipient and donor sites (see Chapter 3); 2% or 4% lignocaine jelly applied to the ulcer for a few moments will often provide adequate anaesthesia for the final preparation of the recipient bed.

Final preparation of the recipient site

The last traces of fibrin and slough should be removed and a clean bleeding bed produced. This can be done by rubbing the granulation tissue with a dry swab or by shaving the granulations using a large scalpel blade or skin graft knife. Bleeding will cease in time if a saline-soaked swab is applied to the bed and left undisturbed while the donor site is prepared. If bleeding remains troublesome, delayed skin grafting after 24 h of firm pressure, dressing and elevation may be advisable.

Pinch grafts (Fig. 8.1)

These are tiny pieces of skin which are full thickness in the middle. They are an alternative to split skin grafts and are most useful in small ulcers over subcutaneous bony areas where a more robust graft is desirable. However, this procedure is a little tedious!

Donor site

The groin provides an excellent donor site. If the grafts are taken from within an ellipse of skin, the donor site can be excised and sutured directly producing a linear scar in a 'hidden' area.

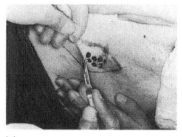
(a)

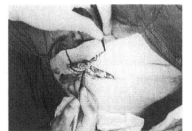
(b)

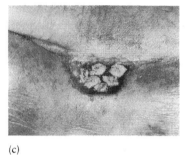
(c)

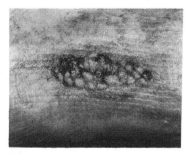
(d)

(e)

Fig. 8.1 (a) Taking pinch grafts from right groin. (b) Excising donor site. (c) Pinch grafts in position on ulcer. (d) Jelonet and cotton wool dressing. (e) Healed ulcer at 12 days.

Technique
1 Local anaesthesia is used to infiltrate the donor area after marking the ellipse.
2 Using a large hypodermic needle, a tiny area of skin is lifted and cut horizontally with a No. 10 or 15 scalpel.
3 The grafts are then applied immediately to the recipient site.
4 The wound is packed with Jelonet and flavine-soaked cotton wool.
5 Firm bandaging should be applied.

Aftercare
A period of elevation and immobilization is desirable for a few hours only.
    The first graft dressing should be at about 7–10 days. This technique produces a slightly more robust graft of 'cobblestone' appearance.

Ingrowing toenails

Surgical treatment

Indication
Chronic, painful ingrowing toenails which have been unresponsive to topical therapy.

Treatment of ingrowing toenails using phenol

Advantages
• Only the lateral ingrowing margin of the nail is removed.
• The lateral matrix is destroyed.
• No incisions or sutures are necessary.
• There is minimal bleeding.
• There is minimal postoperative pain.

Technique
Prior to phenolization, eradicate infection and reduce inflammation, using one of the following.
• Potassium permanganate soaks.
• Topical antiseptics, e.g. Betadine paint.

- Topical antibiotic, e.g. Mupiricin ointment.
- Oral antibiotics (flucloxacillin, amoxycillin).

Phenolization. Insert a ring block, using lignocaine without adrenaline (Chapter 3) and give it time to work (30 min).

Soak and clean the ingrown toenail in an antiseptic solution while the ring block is working (e.g. Hibiscrub solution).

Once the toe is anaesthetized, place a tourniquet around the base of the toe. You can use the glove technique for a toe as well as finger (Chapter 3).

Using English nail splitters, split the nail by inserting the flat blade under the nail adjacent to the lateral ingrowing fragment and cutting down with the upper blade. Continue inserting and cutting until you reach the proximal nail fold. Scissors damage the nail bed and are more difficult to insert. Separate the lateral part of the proximal nail fold from the lateral nail plate gently, using a small flat spatula or septum elevator. Slide the spatula under the fragment of nail to loosen any attachments between the lateral portion of nail and the nail bed.

Grip the lateral fragment of nail with artery forceps and avulse by twisting and pulling.

If necessary, gently curette the lateral nail fold to ensure no fragments of nail are retained.

Smear yellow soft paraffin thickly onto the skin around the nail to protect the nail folds from the phenol.

Twist small wisps of cotton wool onto three orange sticks.

Pour 5 ml of aqueous phenol into a metal dish (*warning*: phenol burns skin and dissolves plastic, so be careful).

Dip the cotton wool tip of the first orange stick briefly into phenol and push into the nail matrix as far as possible. Move the stick around so that the phenol reaches the lateral corner of the matrix. Keep the stick in the matrix for 1 min. Repeat the manoeuvre with the other sticks (1 min/stick).

Immediately wash out the wound thoroughly with alcohol to neutralize the phenol and prevent any more destruction of tissue.

Remove the tourniquet.

Dress with Bactigras or Betadine and Jelonet to provide anti-
sepsis.

Bandage the toe to provide some compression.

Ask the patient to elevate the foot as much as possible for the
next 48 h.

Re-examine the wound after four days or earlier if the patient
has increasing pain.

Complications

1 The chemical burn may induce over-granulation.

2 Normal skin will burn if the phenol splashes or the skin is not
adequately protected.

3 If ablation of the nail matrix is incomplete, a lateral spur of
nail regrows. This does not usually cause symptoms.

4 Infection (rare).

5 Pain, usually minimal.

Acne cysts

Inflammatory cysts respond well to injections of steroids.
Lesions should improve, and possibly drain, within 48 h.

Indication

Palpable, inflamed acne cysts.

Contraindications

Epidermal and pilar cysts ('sebaceous' cysts).

Acne cysts which have drained and cannot be palpated. (If the
steroid does not go into the cyst, the injection may produce
atrophy in the surrounding tissue. Ask the patient to return if the
cyst refills).

Cysts that are not inflamed; these sometimes respond to
cryosurgery.

Technique

Triamcinolone acetonide for injection is available in 5 ml reusable bottles (Lederspan 5 mg/ml). Use a 1 ml insulin syringe with
a fine needle.

No more than 0.25 mg (0.05 ml of triamcinolone 5 mg/ml) should be injected into the middle of the cyst producing slight distension.

You can dilute the triamcinolone to 2.5 mg/ml in saline and inject up to 0.1 ml (0.25 mg) into each cyst.

Chondrodermatitis nodularis chronica helicis

Medical therapy
This is worth trying before surgery, especially in mild cases; it is helpful in about 25% of patients (Lawrence 1991).

Inject 0.2 to 0.5 ml of triamcinolone (10 mg/ml) into surrounding subcutaneous tissue. Apply betamethasone valerate cream twice a day.

Two per cent lignocaine gel should be applied 30 min before going to bed.

Relieve pressure on the ear if possible.

Surgical therapy
Always send the specimen for histological examination.

The ear cartilage must be smoothly contoured after surgery or the condition will recur.

Wedge excision of skin and cartilge: nodules may recur at excision margins where the cartilage is most likely to be irregular.

Cartilage removal alone: a skin flap is raised and the underlying cartilage excised without leaving any protuberant edges. This technique provides a good cosmetic result and it may be easier to smooth the contour of the cartilage (Lawrence 1991).

Further reading
Lawrence, C. (1991) The treatment of chondrodermatitis nodularis with cartilage removal alone. *Archives of Dermatology* 127, 530–535.

Acne keloids
Cryosurgery (Chapter 7): two 15 s freeze–thaw cycles.

Indications
- Keloids less then 6 mm depth.
- Early, more vascular, keloids respond better than older lesions.
- Keloids on the back respond best; keloids on the face respond least well.

Further reading
Layton, A.M., Yip, J. & Cunliffe, W.J. (1994) A comparison of intra-lesional triamcinolone and cryosurgery in the treatment of acne keloids. *British Journal of Dermatology* 130, 498–501.

Medical treatment of pre-malignant skin conditions
Many patients have extensively sun-damaged skin with numerous solar keratoses or multiple areas of Bowen's disease. The clinician should be aware of the medical treatment options available when planning therapy for these patients.

Five per cent Fluorouracil cream (Efudix)
Topical 5% Fluorouracil cream (5-FU) induces brisk inflammation and regression of areas of dysplasia.

Indications
- Numerous solar keratoses.
- Bowen's disease, especially plaques below the knee which may be difficult to excise and close directly. Cryosurgery or radiotherapy to lesions on the leg may produce ulcers which will be slow to heal.

Contraindications
- Squamous cell carinoma (SCC).
- Lesions in which the diagnosis is uncertain. A biopsy should be taken before planning treatment.

Advantages
1 A large area can be treated, including the skin on the face.
2 5-FU does not affect normal skin.
3 5-FU may reveal and eradicate areas of solar keratosis which were not apparent on clinical examination.

4 5-FU may be combined with topical Tretinoin for a more aggressive regime (see below).

Disadvantages
1 Abnormal skin goes red and look unsightly during treatment.
2 Treatment of solar keratoses usually takes two to three weeks; Bowen's disease may take longer to respond.
3 Inflamed skin is uncomfortable near the end of the period of treatment.
4 Patients may continue applying cream although the skin is already very inflamed.
5 Over-treatment with 5-FU may produce ulcers, particularly on the leg.
6 Topical 5-FU may photosensitize the skin, so treatment is most appropriate in the winter.
7 In rare cases, allergic contact dermatitis complicates repeated treatments with 5-FU cream.
8 Solar keratoses and Bowen's disease may recur.

Technique for solar keratoses or Bowen's disease
NB Precise treatment regimes vary.
1 Patients or carers must be able to understand how to apply the cream.
2 The patient should be supplied with written information outlining the plan of treatment.
3 Explain that abnormal skin will become red and uncomfortable during treatment, but the cream will not affect normal skin. Ensure that the patient understands that the skin may look unsightly and that he/she does not have an important social occasion to attend within the next month.
4 Explain that areas of skin that looked normal may also go red because the cream reveals and treats early changes.
5 *Emphasize that the patient must stop treatment once the skin is very red or sore.* This usually takes two to three weeks for solar keratoses but may take longer when treating Bowen's disease.

6 Prescribe 5-FU cream (20 g tube; Efudix) and ask the patient to use gloves when applying the cream.

7 *Solar keratoses*: the patient should apply the cream thinly to all skin in the area to be treated not just the scaly spots, e.g. the face (avoid the eyes), scalp and the forearms.

8 *Bowen's disease*: ensure that the patient includes a 5 mm rim of normal skin when applying the cream to the plaque of disease.

9 Apply the cream once a day for the first week.

10 If the skin is not reacting, the cream should be applied twice a day in the second week.

11 Arrange to review the patient in three weeks so that you can assess the response to treatment.

12 If there is no reaction to 5-FU:
   (a) have you made the right diagnosis?
   (b) has the patient been using the treatment correctly?

Alternative regimes
- Apply 5-FU cream for five days every week and continue until inflamed (this may take four to six weeks).
- Apply 5-FU cream twice a day from the onset of treatment.

After-care
Inflammation and discomfort can be reduced by applying a moderately potent or a potent topical corticosteroid cream twice daily for about one week.

Tretinoin
Tretinoin (a form of vitamin A) may be prescribed as a cream (0.025% Retin A cream). Prolonged use of this preparation may lessen some of the changes associated with sun damage.

Indications
Mild sun damage with solar lentigenes (flat pigmented lesions on sun-damaged skin) and superficial solar keratoses.

Tretinoin may also be prescribed for patients with severely sun-damaged skin prior to using topical 5-FU (see p. 74).

Disadvantages
Tretinoin cream irritates the skin and patients have to build up tolerance to the preparation. Efficacy is limited and it may take 12 months of treatment before improvement is apparent. Topical Tretinoin may cause photosensitivity.

Technique
1 Tretinoin cream (0.025% Retin A cream) is prescribed.
2 The cream is applied thinly to all sun-exposed skin.
3 Initially the patient should apply the cream on alternate days, and gradually the frequency of application is increased to twice a day.
4 Continue treatment twice daily for 8–12 months.
5 After 12 months, reduce the frequency of application to twice weekly.

Technique for severely sun-damaged skin
Patients with widespread solar keratoses and severely sun-damaged skin may respond incompletely to topical 5-FU. If the skin is pre-treated with topical Tretinoin this may improve the efficacy of treatment with 5-FU, but the patient must be warned that the inflammatory response will be severe. The patient must stop treatment when the skin is very inflamed.

Regimen
Months 1–3: Tretinoin cream (0.025% Retin A cream) is applied twice a day to pre-treat the skin.
Month 4: 5-FU cream is applied twice a day until the skin is inflamed (this may take two to six weeks).
   Tretinoin cream may be continued as a midday application for the first two weeks.

Disadvantages
Morbidity is high. Patients may need a brief hospital admission if the skin becomes very inflamed.

Counselling patients

Patients with sun-damaged skin or skin cancers should be advised to avoid the sun when it is at its height, between midday and 3.00 pm. The Mediterranean custom of taking a siesta in the middle of the day makes sense.

Sunshades, tightly woven cotton clothing and broad-brimmed hats protect the skin better than any sun-block cream.

High-factor sun-blocks (factor 15+) will prevent sunburn if applied regularly but should not be used as an excuse to spend more time sunbathing.

Laser surgery

Introduction

The field of laser therapy has advanced rapidly over the last few years; numerous NHS and private facilities have been set up. This section outlines the established uses of lasers on the skin.

The components common to all lasers are shown in Fig. 8.2. Lasers emit a narrow beam of bright light which can travel over long distances without much divergence. Some lasers emit light continuously, while in others the emission is pulsed. Unlike conventional light sources, most lasers have very narrow emission spectra, and the radiation, if in the visible range, is perceived as a pure colour. Some lasers (e.g. argon) have more than one emission peak. The gain medium (e.g. argon, ruby, CO_2) of the laser determines the characteristics of the emitted radiation.

The biological effects of a laser depend on the laser/tissue interactions — these include absorption, scattering and transmission. Tissues vary in their ability to absorb different wavelengths. A red object absorbs all wavelengths except red so that a port wine stain, for example, will absorb a blue-green laser light best. Scattering of photons occurs; the extent is dependant on the particle and the wavelength. The transmission of laser energy through a tissue depends on both absorption and scattering. In a clinical setting a useful concept is the effective penetration depth which is defined as the maximum depth at

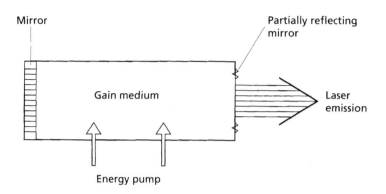

Fig. 8.2 The components of a laser.

which the desired reaction is achievable for a given incident energy. To find the best laser for a given task will, therefore, involve looking at the wavelength that will be absorbed by the target tissue but which is also capable of penetrating deep enough to reach the tissue at sufficient energy levels.

Photothermal and photomechanical reactions
The photothermal reaction indicates that laser energy is converted into heat and is seen with pulsed and continuous dye, copper vapour and argon lasers. Photomechanical effects occur in very short time-scales, e.g. 1 billionth of a second. Very high temperatures are momentarily induced in the target tissue: rather than heat being conducted to surrounding tissues a huge temperature gradient changes into a mechanical shock wave which is capable of fragmenting brittle material, e.g. tattoo pigment. Q-switched ruby and Alexandrite lasers will do this.

Clinical uses

Vascular lesions
Argon lasers have previously been used but thermal energy was conducted through the tissues leading to scar formation in a number of cases. Tunable dye lasers operating at either 577 nm or 585 nm are both effective but each is suited to a different

colour of haemangioma. Moreover they only deal effectively with smaller vessels. Copper vapour and argon lasers with monitored pulse widths are proving useful for larger blood vessels. It can be seen that a range of properties is needed to deal rationally with a port wine stain and at present no single laser fulfills all the needs.

Pigmented lesions
Melanin has a wide absorption spectrum so that most lasers will have some biological effect—but which ones are clinically useful? Pigment is seen at different depths. Red light penetrates deeply but is poorly absorbed by melanin; Q-switched ruby and Neo-dynium YAG lasers seem best suited to the task.

Tattoos
These are similar to pigmented lesions in many respects. Damage is mainly effected by photomechanical interactions. Some tattoo pigment is very deep and can only be reached effectively by the Neodynium YAG laser.

Carbon dioxide laser
This laser has not yet been mentioned because it has such a non-specific thermal effect. It emits infrared radiation which is invisible. A visible light source is incorporated into the machine. Absorption is uniform with minimal scatter and penetration is low.

Uses

Cutting (Light scalpel)
The beam can be focussed into a high-power small spot (0.1–0.2 mm) which causes rapid precise vaporization of tissue and seals blood vessels. The damage is focal because there is almost no heat conducted to the surrounding tissue. It cuts like a scalpel and bleeding is minimal. Excisions, flaps and grafts can all be performed with the CO_2 laser.

Vaporization (Laser abrasion)
If the beam is defocussed, the spot size increases (approximately

2 mm) and is less powerful. It causes localized, superficial, less rapid vaporization of tissue and can be used to plane away layers of tissue or vaporize small tumours, e.g. benign vascular tumours, epidermal naevi and viral warts.

Conclusions

Laser therapy is moving forward quickly. The search for a multi-purpose laser is ongoing but it seems clear that a range of lasers with different wavelengths and pulse widths will be needed for some time. New CO_2 lasers are so precise that skin surface remodelling is possible with benefits similar to that seen after dermabrasion or chemical peels; port wine stain treatment in infants is proving highly satisfactory. The future no doubt holds other extraordinary developments in the field of skin surgery.

Wound Problems

The aim in all surgical endeavours to remove unsightly lesions is to produce thin pale scars which are partly camouflaged by lying in or parallel to natural skin creases. Small, pale, flat, circular scars produced after treatment other than excision may also be relatively unobtrusive. This chapter will outline normal and pathological wound healing with early and late complications of excisional wounds. The prevention and management of these complications will be discussed.

Normal wound healing

If skin edges are accurately apposed, epidermal healing occurs rapidly by bridging across the small blood clot which lies between the wound edges. Granulation tissue develops in the fresh scar and the laying down of collagen in this tissue takes many months to reach a stable state.

It is very important to warn patients that all scars will pass through a phase of being red, indurated and itchy. The degree and length of this process varies from a few months to a year. Eventually a mature, pale, flat scar is produced. Some scars stretch over this period.

Pathological wound healing

Unfortunately some scars remain red and raised (i.e. hypertrophic) for mny months or even years. Keloid scars are those which grow and develop beyond the confines of the original wound. An understanding of the factors which influence ultimate scar behaviour will help both in discussing the outcome of surgery with the patient and in using the best possible technique.

Uncontrollable factors influencing scar behaviour

1 *Age*. Scars in children are generally slower to mature and poorer in the long term. Scars in the elderly seem to settle very quickly.

2 *Site.* Upper chest, upper arms and upper back are notorious for producing hypertrophic, keloidal and stretched scars in susceptible individuals. Scars in these areas may be so ugly that the management of all non-malignant lesions in these areas must be considered very carefully. Stretching of scars also occurs in the mobile skin over joints.

3 *Skin colour.* Dark-skinned individuals and those with red hair tend to produce more hypertrophic and keloidal scars.

Controllable factors influencing scar behaviour

1 *Scar direction.* Skin crease incisions along Langer's lines result in minimal tension across wounds and thus reduce the amount of stretching (see Chapter 5, pp. 32–34).

2 *Wound tension.* Buried dermal sutures will take tension off the epidermis and may reduce scar stretching (see Chapter 5, p. 43).

3 *Suture insertion.* Eversion of wound edges encourages good skin apposition and avoids ugly inverted scars (see Chapter 5, pp. 39–43).

4 *Suture material.* Non-absorbable monofilament nylon sutures produce the least tissue reaction. The finer the suture, the less chance of leaving ugly suture marks.

5 *Timing of suture removal.* Sutures left in for longer than five days will leave suture marks. In areas where it is advisable to maintain wound tension in order to help prevent stretched scars, a subcuticular suture is preferable (see Chapter 5, pp. 42).

6 *Atraumatic technique.* Crushed, avascular tissue leads to the development of more scar tissue and so gentle handling of tissues is vital.

7 *Suture tension.* Similarly, if sutures are too tight, devitalization of the wound edges occurs resulting in more scar tissue and ultimately poorer quality scars.

Early wound complications

Haematoma
The development of a haematoma in any wound is a disaster. It

is likely to become infected and it will lead to excessive fibrosis and a poorer scar. A haematoma may cause the wound to dehisce.

Prevention
1 Meticulous haemostasis prior to wound closure.
2 Closure of any major dead space with deep buried sutures.
3 Application of pressure for a few hours postoperatively where possible.

Treatment
In the small excisions under discussion in this book, small haematomas can usually be left to absorb themselves. Occasionally it may be necessary to open the wound, evacuate the clot and resuture. Sometimes a liquified haematoma can be aspirated.

Infection
Wound infection almost invariably follows the development of a haematoma. It is characterized by increasing redness, pain and swelling in the wound. Discharge of pus through the wound will occur eventually.

Prevention
1 See methods of prevention of haematomas (above).
2 Atraumatic surgical technique.

Treatment
1 Open the wound to allow free drainage of pus by removing one or more sutures.
2 Maintain wound drainage by inserting a small wick of ribbon gauze soaked in aqueous Betadine. Change this dressing regularly until clean.

Wound dehiscence
This is usually secondary to haematoma with or without infection.

Prevention
1 See methods of prevention of haematomas and infection (above).
2 Do not remove sutures too soon (see Chapter 5).
3 Apply Steri-strips to wounds immediately after suture removal if there is concern.

Treatment
Secondary suturing of the wound if it is clean. (NB After secondary suturing, sutures can be removed quite early, i.e. four to five days).

Management of late wound complications

Hypertrophic scars
Massage firmly with emollient cream twice a day and wait for several months.

Hypertrophic and keloid scars
1 Inject with a long-acting steroid (e.g. Triamcinolone). A course of monthly intralesional injections will usually soften up a small keloid in three to six months.
2 Dermovate ointment can be applied under a granuflex dressing and left for six days. A 24 h exposure period of the wound is allowed prior to repeating the treatment. Treatment is carried out for one to two months. Epidermal atrophy is common after prolonged treatment.
3 Superficial radiotherapy is justified only very occasionally. Various other techniques are available. Troublesome keloid scars should be referred to a specialist.

Stretched scars
It may be worth attempting re-excision and suturing with more prolonged wound support. Patients need to be warned that scars will once again pass through a phase of being raised, red and itchy. Specialist advice should be sought.

Further reading

Barron, J.N. & Saad, M.N. (eds.) (1980) *Operative Plastic and Reconstructive Surgery*. Churchill Livingstone, Edinburgh.

McGregor, I.A. (1980) *Fundamental Techniques of Plastic Surgery*, 7th edn. Churchill Livingstone, Edinburgh.

Index